Introducti

Think of a lifesaver, we all need to feel safe and protected.

This book is all about your life and how it will be changed or be made completely new through different aspects of fitness and life tools.

I want to give you a brief description about this book and what you will expect to see. Lifesaver is all about the spiritual, mental, emotional and physical aspects of fitness and how these can apply to our daily lives in knowing how to control certain situations.

I will give you the roadmap to success and help you drop things that are not helping you, like fad diets that don't work. I will take all the guess work out for you, you don't even have to think about preparation.

I will encourage you and tell you about the benefits and struggles of life and how to make sure we get the most out of it.

This life will have ups and downs, that's for sure, but we need to learn that life is a process, and it's all about your journey. If you have fallen down, get right back up and forget about what happened in the past, then move forward.

I know it's just the start of your journey and it's going to be tough. Even so, I know that you have the willpower to do anything.

This process and journey will be hard. It's not a quick fix or putting a temporary Band-Aid on. It's a complete lifestyle change.

So let's move forward and fix what did happen so that the past stops defining us. We will grow stronger in our confidence in ourselves and become the people we were meant to be.

This book will help you find that strong inner person and find out why you are here on this earth. Let's get started.

Do you want a lifesaver?

Table of Contents

Chapter 1 ~ Inner Self 6

    Part 1: Mental 6

    Part 2: Emotional 9

    Part 3: Spiritual 13

Chapter 2 ~ Negative Feed 16

    Negative Feed: 16

Chapter 3 ~ Mental Strength 21

Chapter 4 ~ Sleep/Relief 25

    Sleep: 25

    Relief: 28

Chapter 5 ~ Safety/Form 30

    Form: 30

    Safety: 32

Chapter 6 ~ Calories/Breakfast 35

    Calories: 35

    Breakfast: 37

Chapter 7 ~ Motivation 40

Chapter 8 ~ Hydration 45

Chapter 9 ~ Carbs/Fats/Protein 49

    Protein: 49

- Carbs: 51
- Fats: 52

Chapter 10 ~ Exercise Program 54
- FITNESS: 54
- Exercise Types: 55
- Cardio: 55
- Strength: 56
- Strength with Dumbbells: 58
- Yoga: 59
- Abs/Core: 59

Chapter 11 ~ God's View of Fitness 61

Chapter 12 ~ Food Journal 66

Chapter 13 ~ Drinking and Smoking 69

Chapter 14 ~ Body Obsession 72

Chapter 15 ~ Treat Day/Cheat Day 74

Chapter 16 ~ Judgment/Attitude 79

Chapter 17 ~ Pain And Hurts 85

Chapter 18 ~ Forgive Yourself And Forgive Others 92

Chapter 19 ~ Healthy Meal Plan/Recipes 98
- Breakfast: 98
- Lunch Menu: 103

Chapter 20 ~ Exercises 108

Core Stability Training: 108

Cardiovascular Interval Training 123

Strength Training... 126

Stretches and Yoga Poses: 138

Workout Plan: 148

Chapter 21 ~ Myths of Fitness 149

Chapter 22 ~ Benefits/Tips on Fitness 156

5 Main Benefits of Healthy Nutrition.......................... 161

Closing ~ Lifesaver.. 164

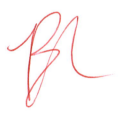

Chapter 1 ~ Inner Self

You were created mentally, emotionally, and the most important: SPIRITUALLY.

These integral parts of humanity play a huge part in our fitness goals and in life. When you focus on the inner self, the outward appearance will be reflected. Are you feeling better? Why?

It's probably because of a change in your daily life because the inner self is more important than anything else.

We have to learn how to KO those unwanted and unnecessary comments, feelings, and negativity. Getting them out of your system will lead to a happier and healthier life that we all deserve.

Part 1: Mental

When it comes to the basics of life, what helps us remember our daily emotions?

The answer is the way we communicate, function and express ourselves to others around us. Our brains are an important part of keeping us alive and well.

In this chapter I will explain why mental training in fitness is so important. First, I will ask a question, why do you think your brain is important to you?

You may think the answer is mathematic skills, social skills, communication, etc; you get the point. Fitness was created to help you have a better understanding of how the human body works.

We have doctors, scientists, trainers, massage therapists and physiotherapists that study and analyse the human body.

The body is so important and we need to understand that there is a science behind every aspect of life. We need to learn how the body functions and maneuvers.

What is the first thing you think about when it comes to fitness? Is it those dumbbells or the treadmill? Here is the definition of fitness: it is the capability of the body to distribute inhaled oxygen to the muscle tissue during increased physical effort.

Fitness is about breathing in a controllable way to deliver oxygen to the muscles. Fitness is about breathing control, which is a very mental thing.

Your mind is such an important part of your workouts because it plays an 80% role in your goals. If you commit to a realistic goal, you can attain it.

When you are working out, you need to focus on the movements your body is making so you can improve and strengthen the muscles without getting injured.

For example: if you are doing a squat, you need to listen to my instructions so that you don't get hurt.

Here's the form for a squat: hips back towards the wall, chest up so I can see your head, back flat, knees behind your toes.

Just try it, getting form right takes mental effort. It's just as mental as it is physical, emotional, or spiritual.

If you come to a trainer and say: "I want to get in shape, or lose weight." There's a mental reason why you came in the first place and it isn't all about the weight loss.

There's a drive in you that wants something to improve. It happens more than you can recognize. You need to make a change but sometimes you don't know where to start.

That's where I come in. As a trainer, I want everyone to live happier and healthier, but I can't do anything until you make a choice to say, "I'm ready for a life changer inside."

When I put that realistic goal together for you, I expect you to be mentally ready to dig deep inside your head and break through the thoughts that were telling you that you can't do it.

I'll be there saying that I believe in you. I genuinely know you can do this. I'll be your counsellor, friend and coach to help you and motivate you to keep up the good effort and say you're worth it.

I know that you can do anything when you put your mind to it. That seems like a childish answer, but I am really saying that you can do anything you set your mind to.

Focus on your goal and start by taking little baby steps to get there. Let me tell you something, there are people in this world that will tell you that you can't do anything. But what about Albert Einstein, Benjamin Franklin, Bill Gates, Robin Williams, Tom Cruise, Walt Disney.

All of these guys had a learning disability. But they didn't give up when the world told them it was hopeless for them to pursue a well-educated career. Look at them now.

They are some of the most famous people in the world. My point is, no matter where you are on your fitness journey, you can push through any obstacle in life and learn how to work around it.

I know you are mentally capable of so much more than what you think you can do. I believe with all my heart you are worth it and my first tip is: don't let negative people bring you down, look in that mirror and be the best friend and best encourager.

Every day that you look in the mirror, say I love you for being yourself and you can do anything you set your mind to.

Part 2: Emotional

Let's talk about the emotional side of fitness, and how it applies to your daily life today. Let's talk about the reason why you are reading this book, and why you came to have an understanding about your emotional habits.

First, let's talk about how your emotions play a part in fitness. When you are working out and you have a certain feeling inside, it's healthy to let it out.

When you are stressed out at work or mad at a family member, let all your frustration out in that gym and leave it there. It's not healthy to carry baggage around with you, you need to let it go and get it off your back.

Fitness will teach you that when your muscles are burning and you need to push through it, scream, shout and get all that pain out of your body because you deserve it.

You are valuable and you earned the right to be happy and enjoy life. Don't let your past define you, and leave those unwanted pains and sorrows behind you.

Find a close person, and tell them about your struggles and problems; a friend, family member, trainer.

You will feel so much better once you let it go. I know I have been through so much in my life, from when I was a kid until now.

I held hatred toward certain people because of the pain they gave, but as I grew up, people could see my pain, and I realized I couldn't deal with this anymore.

My friend took me to the gym and I went in there as a sad person, and came out radically transformed and happy.

I learned that I'm not the only person who has been through so much; I realized I could get through it with the help and support of my friends who encouraged me and helped me out.

Through my experience I gained faith, and believe that when you are crying and get mad in the gym, you need to leave all those unwanted emotions that you are carrying, and become a newly transformed person.

Next I want to say there is a deep heart issue when fitness and emotions that comes hand and hand and play a huge part in your current life now.

Sometimes we might have wounds or hurts that we don't know of. You know what I'm talking about when you get emotional and don't understand why you're sad or upset about.

That is a big problem we need to fix and get to the bottom of. It could have been you were abused as a kid, bullied at a young age, might not have remembered, but your emotions remember the whole situation.

It's sad, but we need to learn how to deal with them in a healthy manner. That's why when I am working out with a client I need to know why they came to me in the first place.

I'll give you an example: Once I see them in action in the gym and I see they can't go past their barrier or push past their comfort level.

There needs to be something changing here, because something's not adding up. If I tell you to GO HARD and Dig Deep and then you stop, why are you stopping and why did you come to me in the first place if you're not ready.

There has to be a heart issue behind the workout, that's where the emotion side comes out, tell your trainer what's going on and he/she might encourage you to go beyond the limits and forgive yourself and forgive those people who hurt you.

What happened is history and we can push through the pain and get over to the over side and feel accomplished and renewed that you can do anything once you renew your mind and take control over your emotions and release those pains in the workout and forgive.

It's key to have a plan and use your life experiences to Forgive and Overcome and start to take small steps to get you to your realistic goal.

When you want to feel better about how you look you need to stand face to face to reality and accept yourself for who you are in the first place.

Next step after that is to say to yourself I AM READY TO CHANGE. Don't let people get in your way towards getting the best body you always dreamed of.

You need to tune them out and say I don't care about what people say I am or who I used to be, I care about who I say I am, and not rely on who people say I am. I am my own best friend and my own worst enemy.

You need to learn how to control the emotional side and not let it take control over your life. You are in control of every aspect of your life.

Part 3: Spiritual

Lots of people don't believe there is a spiritual side to fitness, most of this world doesn't want to think that your inner self has a soul or spirit, but you have inner voices that speak to you and tell you words.

When I was getting certified, my teacher told me that there is a spiritual side to fitness, but she didn't really talk much about that side or even want to discuss it, because she didn't really believe in the spiritual side of fitness and how it comes into play.

There are four aspects of fitness: Physical, emotional, mental and spiritual. Your spirit is your inner person and you need to help take control of it.

The way I love to get in tune with my spirit is through yoga, stretches, and meditation. I want to start with Yoga: Yoga started in the eastern culture and was used for religious purposes.

As it transferred from Eastern to Western Culture is seemed to lose it spiritual value. We just treated it as if it was nothing, just working out to stretch and relax.

That is part of your Yoga practice, but that's not all of it. Yoga is a way to get inside and connect with your inner self. Tap into your soul and recharge, calm it down from the stress.

When I do Yoga, sometimes I feel sleepy and rested because it is the time for me to get out all those hard obstacles from family or work, and just calm down.

Yoga is created to help you rest, relax and get rid of any anxiety or stress. When I do Yoga, I love to focus on my spirit and mind and tune everything else out.

Because you don't need to think about anything other than yourself. If you want to help others, you need to help yourself first.

Then once you're in tune and up to date and reach your peak point, then you will start to serve and help others out. I believe God uses yoga to speak to his children in a way to focus on what he has blessed us with, and be thankful for what he has given to you.

When you think and focus on those positive thoughts while you're doing yoga poses and exercise, it's a time for you to thank God for blessing you with all you have in your life.

In the fitness and exercise section of this book you will see some yoga poses like the mountain pose and corpse pose. I love to do these poses because it shows you how to control your breathing and focus on your body, mind and spirit.

Take care of your spirit and treasure it. Your spirit is valuable, and plays a big part in your life. You deserve it. Your inner self is just as important as your outward appearance. Whatever is happening on the inside is a reflection of the outward appearance.

This is the key to understanding your own spirit, having a connection to fitness, and letting your whole body connect and work together.

You can control and focus on your own body alignment. Once you let your mind, body and soul come together there is no stopping you from achieving your fitness goal.

Chapter 2 ~ Negative Feed

Negative Feed:

If something looks impossible or hard we automatically say "I can't do that." Why do you think we talk like this? Is it because of negative surroundings, other people, or media?

What we need to do is to reprogram our mental tape and start recording new words, saying "I can, believe in myself, I'm worth it."

I would suggest not to go alone when wanting to try something that you haven't done before so don't go alone. Get a support group.

Go to group fitness classes to help encourage one another and build yourself up. Slowly, one by one, start knocking out negative words and start filling your vocabulary with positive words.

As humans we are full of negative feedback. Negative news is everywhere, but we need to think positive.

Here's an exercise, I have two columns, the first one filled with positive words, and the second filled with negative words.

We need to be the person who can turn a negative feed into positive feed. Step one: every time you say a negative word to yourself or someone else, drop and do ten push-ups right away.

Sounds good, but it's going to be hard. It's a process. Don't let people turn you the wrong way. Listen to my instructions, and I will help you along this stage of your journey.

We all have been there, and said something bad about others. It's a bad habit that needs to get broken. Forgive yourself for everything that has happened to you, and what people have done to you.

You have carried all that baggage for a long time. Down below write positive and negative comments that you say about yourself.

Post this list on your fridge, so you can stay motivated to know everyday is a struggle and process and we all need encouragement.

Positive Comments	Negative Comments

Next we are going to talk about why you get these thoughts, and how to get rid of them.

Have you been physically or emotionally hurt by someone? What do you think happens after all of that has occurred in your life? Do you want revenge? Do you just hide or run away?

Name the first problem you have dealt with: _____
_____

How did it make you feel upset, frustrated, sad, depressed, or anxious?

Once you know how you felt about it, then we have a starting point. Was it a poor choice? Or did you learn to deal with it in a proper and healthy manner.

Example: Say you got bullied at school one day and the kid punched you and it hurt you physically and you cried.

How did you deal with it, frustration? Did you want to beat him up? This is the wrong motive. Learn to stand up for yourself and say to him, "I'm sorry for all the tragedy that has happened to you."

Say, "I forgive you for everything you have done," it's hard to say it, but I guarantee that you will feel better about yourself and learn to deal with it better next time.

Talking gets to the root of the problems, not fighting. First of all, recognize the emotions you are facing at that period of time. Second, learn to act in a loving way and see how they respond and act back towards you or others.

Point three, just forgive, even if it isn't your fault. Lastly, love them as a friend, and don't treat them differently.

Love is the key to success in life and fitness. These are the four points to help you deal with negative thoughts that come into your head and learn to react in the opposite spirit.

Once you grab a hold of that action remember it, and don't forget what I told you. Love upon others and walk in the unexpected loving spirit.

It will change the way you come in contact with others. Let me show you a fitness point of view about this NEGATIVE FEED, when I put you on a treadmill, what do you think about? "I hate this treadmill," I love this treadmill ".

Understand why you feel a certain way about a certain piece of equipment or tool. Why does it make you feel mad, sad or upset? Sometimes we will get confused, or mad, because we are scared of change.

We need to let go of fear and learn that the treadmill is here to change your body and sculpt your life for the better.

Once you learn the science of the body and why you function and move, it will transform every aspect of life from negative thoughts to emotional reactions.

You need to change your way of thinking towards fitness equipment. If you haven't used it before, don't judge until you have experienced it.

Negative feed only has power over your life when you dwell on it and let it take control over you.

Tip: don't dwell on negative words or comments.

Focus on the love of God and love from people around you. This is a huge topic that we need to learn, how to deal with emotions in the right way, and talk about the negative talk going around, before it gets out of hand.

As your trainer writing this book, I want to encourage you to never give up hope on anything even if it seems hopeless. There is a light on the other side, even if you can't see it.

If you believe you will get through that tough part of your life, it will change, and you will become a new person that is totally transformed. Give change time.

Anything you need or want takes time. We need to learn that time can work with us or against us. Time will come around the corner, and before you know it, you will get to the place you always wanted to be.

Chapter 3 ~ Mental Strength

When you're working out, don't just swing the weights around, you have to think about what you are doing.

For example: when you do a bicep curl, you have to put your mind into your workout and think about your biceps. Try to understand a full body workout. It all starts when your head is in the game.

Your whole body has to be in sync. Use both mental and physical strength next time you are in the gym. It will increase your strength and you will have a better overall performance.

I know that I have been talking about mental strength a lot, but again, over 80% of a workout is mental strength. You have to focus on your goals in the gym and avoid getting distracted because of people or things around you.

That's why you don't give up when it seems too hard. Once you put your mind to the test, everything else will make much more sense and you will have better results.

You need to understand that when you want to get the career you want it is relatively easy to get that high position to become a manager or business owner. It takes time and lots of work to be a successful business owner/manager.

We tend to put fitness in a different category than life. We think of fitness as difficult and too much effort and time.

You need to put the effort in to play with the kids, energy to work, and endurance to keep going on a project. Fitness is a life-changing process.

That's why we call it a PROCESS or a JOURNEY. Fitness sculpts and shapes your life. It changes your mindset; how you look at yourself in the mirror, the way you look at others and how you value life.

If you wouldn't have started this journey you probably wouldn't be reading this now. Fitness is more than the gym; it's about how you feel about yourself in the daily situations you face.

Fitness is about how you value things about your new life now. Fitness gives you a second chance to live the life you wanted to live. No more hiding.

It's time to roll up your sleeves and show yourself how much you deserve to enjoy a life full of joy, happiness and wonder. During this experience I want you to remember how you felt the first day of working out, and never forget that feeling.

Use that as motivation to never go back to the old self who felt awful about themselves but now feel like they are living life like it should be. So go explore this world in your new life and new body.

You will thank me later once you are running up those mountains and seeing beautiful nature without getting winded up the hill. Fitness is hard for a reason, to show you that you need to work hard mentally if you really want something in this life.

Nothing comes easy, so the logic is that if you need to pursue something with all your heart I guarantee that you will succeed in your goals.

Now you are making the first step to start your program and get back on track and on the path to success.

I will guide you and give you helpful tips and rules in the directions of losing weight, toning up and getting in shape.

My point is that when you think, and put your mind to the muscles' position, you can push longer than just doing it without thinking.

I know from experience and from my clients that it can have an impact on how you think about your body, mind and life.

Mental strength is one of the most **IMPORTANT PARTS OF FITNESS.**

Don't ever go into a gym thinking you know everything. You can always learn something new, just as the old saying goes, you learn something new every day.

I know you will be surprised and shocked about the history and knowledge that comes into play with sports and fitness science, as well as nutrition and vitamin studies. It will get you thinking about how your body, mind and soul are greater than we can comprehend.

Researchers are still discovering more minerals, cells and muscles in the body do this every day. We don't know everything about the body, but it is mind blowing how little we know about our bodies, and how complex it is put together.

Learn about your body, because we are all different inside and out. We all react to different foods and exercise in different ways. Never count yourself out of the game.

Chapter 4 ~ Sleep/Relief

Sleep:

Sleep has a big effect on your workout. If you don't have enough sleep, you can't give an exercise your all.

You should get an average eight hours of sleep a day. Also, avoid getting too much sleep, as too much sleep will make you feel overly tired or sleepy during the day.

And don't get less than 8 hours of sleep, otherwise you can't function at 100% in the gym. You may think results just come from nutrition and working out, but the top three aspects for changing your fitness are: nutrition, exercise and sleep.

Sleep is the time to let our muscles rest and relax from the hard day you put them through. It's a time to loosen up.

Sometimes we need to take a nap during the day to recharge the system and have more energy. Your energy level can determine how much rest you get from the past night.

Healthy snacks and activities are also very important. If you feel sleepy, try having a handful of nuts to give you some energy.

Sometimes it is hard to fall asleep. When we dwell on work and stress in the evening, this can cause problems in the night.

If you are overweight, sometimes you might have sleep apnea which is a sleeping disorder. A sleep apnea machine is a machine that will breathe for you if you're struggling to sleep.

During the night, if you can't breathe on your own, this machine kicks in and helps you breathe. This may be a very risky move, because I wouldn't want a machine keeping me alive instead of controlling my own breath and health.

The two types of people who may use a sleep apnea machine may have physical problems with their weight, or are sometimes lazy. We need to fight for our life and not have people or machines focus for us and do all the work.

If you don't absolutely need the machine, don't use it! Our bodies are meant to heal themselves through rest and sleep.

Studies have proven that if you have strokes, diabetes, hypertension, or heart disease you will have more difficulty getting good sleep. This will result in more stress.

Ask yourself these questions, and if any of these apply to you in this book, you may need help to focus on your fitness and nutrition goals and help you sleep and recover faster so you can get back to your normal state of sleeping and daily life.

Consult with your doctor before starting any fitness or nutrition plan. As a trainer I care about you and your living situation, and I am here to give you advice and help.

Sleep is something we need because we can't go for days without crashing and burning out. You need to take care of your body and rest when it is time to rest.

No person can tell you how much rest or recovery time your body needs to function. Only you can say, "I need to take some recovery time to get back to my normal state."

It's a mental battle where you need to sit down and think; "how can I change my sleeping pattern to help my overall health and well-being?"

Do you snore when you sleep, or have pauses between breaths when you sleep? Do you have difficulty staying asleep? Do you use a sleep apnea machine? Does sleepiness or fatigue happen when you wake up so you can't function normally?

These are question to ask your doctor. Consult with your physician about any sleeping patterns that you need to change, then make a change.

There is only one way to go, and that is up. Slowly but surely, you will start to feel better and sleep better. It's not going to happen overnight. It will take time.

Remember, there is no finish line. You will feel much better once you include nutrition and fitness into this program, then change will start to kick in. You will slowly start to feel a little difference in your body.

That means you are getting healthier and stronger. It's your journey, fight your fight, and don't fall by the wayside. Trainer Braydon is here for you.

Relief:

Relief is a term used for relaxation. In fitness this would be a rest day. Once a week we need to have some down time and not do anything. It's okay to have a lazy day.

I love sitting around sometimes and doing nothing. If I work hard for six days in a week, I deserve to have that one day to relax, get relief and just calm down.

Never workout seven days a week because you will burn out and you will not be able to recuperate and replenish your body and get it back in order so you can have the strength for another week. Rest is so important; rest is the time when muscles and joints rebuild.

That is the one day I don't have to worry about getting exhausted in a workout. I just say yes to no burn today.

Your rest day is key towards getting the body you always wanted. Sometimes your body can go into shutdown mode and not respond the way you want it to because it hasn't had the rest it needs.

It's like a kid, if they don't want to eat their veggies they will keep their mouth closed and wait for the candy or McDonald's instead.

The human body is smart enough to know what it can handle and what can be used for fuel. If you don't give your body enough sleep, relief, or rest, it might not function at its best, or the way you want it to.

We are so confused and misled, because different people tell us that we are doing right, when only some of it is true.

Scientists are researching how people can get a rest with or without a rest period. This can be risky. Just because you chug protein powder doesn't mean your body is getting what it needs.

Yes, protein helps rebuild muscle tissue, but it might cause your body to go into overdrive, and there might be an incorrect signal reading in your body if you don't give it what it needs. Relief and rest are good to do.

If you are a person who likes to be active all the time, I would recommend you to buy a massage roller and do active stretches on your rest day.

It will help you to relax your innermost deep tissue muscles, and it will reduce your soreness level. You will feel better when you do a deep tissue massage, and it will calm you down.

Whether your rest day is Sunday or Wednesday, take it. If you want to get maximum results in the right amount of time I guarantee your success if you take proper rest.

Your goals will happen if you listen to my instructions on nutrition and fitness plans.

Chapter 5 ~ Safety/Form

Form:

When you are working out, form is the most important thing. If you don't do it right, there's no point in doing any exercise in the first place.

When you do a certain exercise, make sure that your body alignment is perfect. Make sure your knees don't go past your toes during a squat.

Correct form prevents injuries and reduces soreness in the body. Remember, exercising is about strengthening a certain body part. No pain or injuries should occur.

Be wise when doing exercises. Keep correct technique when you're working an isometric muscle group. Never give up, keep it going.

When we are in the gym sometimes we get distracted by another person or object. We need to learn not to get distracted when we're in the gym or at home working.

Distractions can lead to injuries and joint problems in the body. Form is one of the most important elements of exercise. Even though my clients want me to do the work, I'm like you, I need to learn how to do the exercises right.

You need to know how to do the exercise alone for when I'm not around. Say you do some exercises at home, or you go on a hiking adventure. You need to make sure you are doing the activity safely and wisely.

The last thing you want to do is twist yourself in the wrong direction. I'm not there if you forgot the proper form for certain exercises like single leg squats, lunges or even plyometric moments.

That's why form is the most important element to me, because it helps with strengthening the body while working on posture, flexibility and much more.

Bad form leads to torn muscles or broken bones – and that hurts. That's why I want to keep you from looking around at what other people are doing.

Instead, focus on your own workout and how your body is aligned. If you're holding an isometric pose, don't twist any body part because you might hear weird sounds or cracks that aren't supposed to happen.

Just focus on the moment and listen to what your body is telling you. Listen so that you personally know how you feel. How are your muscles feeling? Are they burning or aching? Are bones cracking?

You know your body better than anyone else, so you need to know your own limits and learn when you have pain in your joints because of bad form or technique.

An important part of form is that you need to keep your breath in control. In daily life, do you ever hold your breath? If you're lifting heavy things at work, do you hold your breath? If not, why do you hold it when it comes to stretches, weight training and abs?

Breathing is an important part of form and technique. When you breathe naturally or continuously, you will improve your repetitions, and your form will be perfect.

Here is a tip before you take your workout to the next level of intensity, make sure your form is correct and your body is properly aligned.

Form is the master in fitness. Form first, then speed and then intensity. Safety comes first, if your form is going out the window, but your speed is up, stop and correct the movement to make sure you know how your body alignment is.

I don't care if you can get more reps with bad form, I would rather you do less reps with good form than many reps with bad form.

Form and safety is the most important part of the workout. I know you've heard it a lot, but sometimes when you read or hear something again, you remember it and get better results in the programs you are doing now.

Safety:

When you first start a fitness or exercise program you need to know how to work out safe so you don't hurt yourself. You need to work hard and wisely.

Safety is more important to me than anything else. I would rather you understand the exercise before jumping right in and tearing a muscle.

Safety and form come first, then digging deep and getting uncomfortable. You need to make sure you take care of your body and listen to it when it is in pain.

Safety is important in any aspect of life.

We need to be careful when we walk the streets. In the same way, when you do bodily training like Olympic lifting you need to use the right equipment to make sure not to tear a muscle or break a bone.

You can use different tools to make sure you stay safe in a workout. A safe workout makes it harder to make excuses not to workout.

You can use knee braces, ankle supports, hip belt supports, back braces, arm bands, etc. There are more than these few safety tools that help with form, safety, and technique.

These fitness tools are a lifesaver. If we didn't have them we would have so many more bad backs, broken knees, and twisted ankles than we do today.

I am thankful for all the equipment and accessories that we have to protect our bodies. It is not safe to go into a gym without knowing how to use any of the equipment.

My opinion is to get an orientation of the gym and learn how to use everything correctly, so that you come back knowing how to use the equipment.

Take notes and write it down or type it in your phone. Don't be afraid to ask any question or comments to your trainer about a certain way he does a routine or action. Ask questions all the time.

It's your body, and you need to know if you're doing exercises correctly. Gym courtesy is also important for the sake of safety.

Never leave dumbbells or barbells on the floor; people could trip on them and hurt themselves. Keep your area clean and be aware of your surroundings.

Chapter 6 ~ Calories/Breakfast

Calories:

Calories are a big thing in our everyday life. What I want you to do is to think about the difference between bad and good calories.

What is a bad calorie? Saturated fat, sodium, fat, deep fried foods and fast food. What are the Good Calories?

They are fresh veggies and fruit, whole wheat pastas, lean meat, and proteins like chicken, beef and turkey. If you are vegetarian or vegan there are options like tofu, quinoa, tempeh, Greek yogurt, and veggie burgers.

You need to think about what you are putting inside your system. Ask yourself one question. Is this food going to satisfy me in the long run?

We are usually on a tight time frame and don't care about food preparation. We care about money and appointments, and make sure we are on time.

What we need to do is make time in our day to prepare good, healthy foods and store them for later.

When it is time to work, you have all your food prepared ahead of time. All you have to do is grab that plastic container full of healthy meals and head out on your way.

It's just as simple as our mothers told us: eat your veggies and go outside and play. Not, fill your body up with crap that won't satisfy you in the long run.

There is a time and place to have a splurge meal even on this life saver program. There are rules and guidelines, but this will help you to stay on track if you add a treat meal into your daily routine.

We will talk more about that later. Calories in and calories out doesn't always cut it. It works for some people, but for others it's a discouragement.

What you need to do is learn different methods of calorie counting and learn to read the food labels on the back of the package.

Just because you grab a can of corn doesn't mean that its 1 serving, it could be 4 servings. I'll teach you what to look for in labels and tell you if it's worth the extra time and effort to read and feel better, or grab in a rush and feel awful afterwards.

Breakfast:

I want to talk about the most important meal of the day, which is breakfast. This is a topic that I want to talk about because it has a huge impact on your fitness and nutrition goals.

There is a reason why it is called the most important meal of the day. After you have had at least 8 hours of sleep you need to break the fast, since you were sleeping for a while, and now your body is craving fuel to function through the day.

Here are some food ideas you can try: oatmeal, fruits, veggies, and smoothies. If you want to get the most out of your day, you need energy to do it; to do paperwork, deal with clients, or work on a project.

You need the right amount of food in your system so you can give it your all and fill up for the day. I guarantee that if you beat the clock you can get a good healthy nutritious breakfast.

If you need to work at 7:30am take out a plastic container of fruit, then drive to work. How much time do you need to eat? Set your alarm clock a few minutes back so you can have a good day. Want to do something with someone who is new?

You start small, with a small choice like eating an apple and yogurt for breakfast. Once this is part of your life, then it will be a lot more natural to eat in the morning.

What do most people who have great weight loss success have in common? They eat breakfast, exercise, and drink lots of water. This is all proven by scientists, and clients such as yourself.

Breakfast will be your first step towards a healthy life. Don't change everything at once. All I want you to do is eat breakfast and look at some of my nutrition plans. There will be plenty of choices to eat healthy and make it taste like heaven.

Next subject I want to talk about is counting calories. It's hard work at first to learn how to count calories, but once you learn to train your eye to know what a serving size looks like, then you won't have to use measuring cups and tablespoons as much.

My advice is to count every calorie you insert into your body. Once you know how much you consume everyday then it will get easier for you to know how many calories are in a package or serving size.

You've heard it all before, but I'm going to say it again. Breakfast is the most important meal of the day.

Many people are going through their day not eating breakfast, but what they don't know is that a great day starts in the morning and eating breakfast can help you focus and function better through the day and help you concentrate better.

Breakfast should be eaten within 30-45mins of waking up. Also, once you wake up drink a glass of water right away to get your metabolism revved up and moving for the day.

It's like an old car in the winter that you need to start and warm up to get the engine moving. Once it's warm, it can do its task of transporting people to places.

That's how your metabolism works, you need to hydrate it to give it a kick-start like the key in the ignition.

Breakfast and water will kick start your morning to give you a happy and great day.

Tip: Drink at least 4 - 8oz of water in the morning before and after breakfast.

Chapter 7 ~ Motivation

One of the most asked question is "how do I stay motivated?" Well I'm going to tell you, motivation is hard for everyone, even me.

I've made this book to help you stay motivated and keep you on track. I'm here to help you and keep you going.

You can get a support group, or get your friends or family involved in what you're doing to help you to stay on track, and encourage one another to meet your fitness goals.

Motivation is all about supporting and changing yourself from the inside out; to transform that heart of yours, and make a difference spiritually, physically, mentally and emotionally.

So let's all get on board and help motivate everyone to change their lifestyle one rep at a time. How do I stay motivated?

Well the first week is easy; I feel good about what I'm doing. But how do I keep the rhythm going? I'm going to tell you how to keep on going, even when it starts to get hard.

First: remember how hard it was the first moment when you stepped foot into the gym? You struggled and almost gave up hope on this journey of yours.

You need to remember how you felt and how you don't want to go back to that old lifestyle anymore.

Then you will make a change in your life. There is no finish line in the fitness industry.

There will be ups and down when it comes to your weight loss goal or toning goals. You say "well you're a trainer Braydon and you love to work out and eat healthy."

News flash, the reason why I keep doing what I'm doing is because I'm not perfect, I continue to educate and gain knowledge about the human body and mind.

I worked my butt off to get where I am today. I didn't always love to be active, sometimes I want to be lazy. Sometimes I don't like eating healthy.

It's a journey and a process. Life is tough, but we need to learn to face our situation head on. Keep your head up and learn to fight for this one and only life you have. Treat your life with respect and love.

I don't care what others say about what you look like or act like, it does not matter. I want you to love yourself and care about who you are on the inside.

Here's a question: who lives in this body? That person beside you, your family member or a friend? Do they move your limbs or breathe for you? The answer is no.

I can't do anything but motivate you and show you an alternate route to help you feel better about your inner self and outward appearance.

I am here to help you understand that NO HUMAN can say you are WORTHLESS. If someone tells you that, it's because they have inner problems and don't know how to deal with it or don't want to admit they have any problems.

They are looking for a temporary fix by putting it off on others or picking on people and hoping it will make them feel better for the short term, and their pain will hopefully leave.

I want to give you long term success, not short term. The way I can give you long term success is by helping you through your reasoning, discovering why you came to me in the first place, and why you wanted to start a fitness route.

Ask the question: why do you do New Year's Resolutions and then quit? If you don't finish, what's the point of starting in the first place.

I am here to enter the deep roots of why you care so much about your health. I am not just going to be your personal trainer, I'm going to be your fitness counselor and mentor.

The outward appearance is a reflection of what is going on in the inside. If you look sad a lot, don't have your weight under control, are frustrated all the time, and people can see that you emotionally and mentally struggle, even if you deny it, the human body can show proof of it.

You can tell through an emotion if someone is okay or not. Fitness doesn't just change the physical body; it changes the structure of your life. Change your view on how you act towards people, and how you value your life.

Motivation is key towards getting the best life. Motivation is about transforming your emotions, mind and spiritual soul inside you.

These 3 aspects have an impact on your daily life: fitness and motivation is about supporting and encouraging people through our daily motions.

We need to talk about it the unwanted or confused emotions and get the emotion out of the body that is unwanted.

Motivation is about trusting and committing that you will do whatever it takes to become a better human being. You need to want to live the life that you were created to live, not live a messed up life.

Learn from your mistakes and turn the corner where the grass is greener and life is full of fun, joy and happiness. It will fill you up and make you new. The simple formula for motivation leads you to a new place that will create a new you with new habits and new goals to a new life.

Don't forget that this will take the rest of your life and you need to know that there isn't a finish line. We all mess up and fall flat on our face. All we have to do it get back up.

If you have fallen once or 100 times, you keep getting back up and don't let the past mistakes define you because you are overcoming or have overcome hurdles in your life.

Motivation is the action or reason to react in a certain way. If you're motivated to eat better, you will focus on changing your eating habits.

Motivate yourself with the most important parts of what your life is about. Motivation will keep you on track to getting a better life, and improving on it, for the rest of your life.

Chapter 8 ~ Hydration

Drinking water is one of the most important things you should do throughout the day to keep the body and mind functioning properly.

You should drink at least 7-11 glasses of water per day or half of your body weight. Say you weigh 150lbs, you then divide that in half, which is 75 lbs.

Then move the decimal to the left. This would equal 7.5oz, which is how much water to drink in a day. Listen to your body when it comes to hydration, the last thing you want to be is dehydrated.

These are just guidelines to help you but first and foremost you need to listen to how your body functions with water.

How are you feeling now? Are you hungry, thirsty, or full? You know your body better than anyone else.

Here is the most important thing I want to tell you about hydration or fluid intake: you need to make sure that when you wake up every morning start the day off right by drinking glasses of water to stay hydrated and keep your system running for the day. Take care of your body and the environment.

Many times, we mentally tell ourselves that we are hungry all the time. Next time you are in the office going for those doughnuts, try this test to make sure you're hydrated.

Drink a large glass of water and see if you are still hungry. There is a good chance that you are not hungry anymore. It is boredom and habit that makes us grab food and put it in our mouth without thinking.

There's a good chance that when you grab food when you are not hungry and it is not a meal time, you are actually dehydrated and need to drink more water.

Next time you see yourself looking for those chips or doughnuts in the office, check if you are truly hungry or are just stress eating or eating because you are bored.

Make sure you watch your eating because you might react without thinking. Next time you see yourself grabbing for food, think, when was the last time you had a meal then ask yourself how much water you had today.

If the answer is that you only had four glasses of water in the last six hours you need to get more water and keep your body hydrated. You need to stay awake and functioning on your tasks.

Here are some cool tips about water: did you know that drinking water can help with your skin complexion? It can keep your skin looking smooth and tight.

Next tip: did you know when you're a kid your metabolism is fast, but when you get older it slows down.

The reason is because your body is in the stage of building your figure as a child and once you get older it slows down, especially when you don't take care of it.

We all need to drink two or three glasses of water in the morning to get the metabolism running and burning fat and calories and keep the body lean and tight.

Water is a miracle liquid because you can drink it without worrying about the calories in it unless you add flavors.

Make sure you don't drink from disposable water bottles because they contain unwanted and unnecessary chemicals that are not supposed to be in your body.

Did you know that disposable bottle lids are not fully tightened, so anything can get inside when they are in the store?

It seems like the lid is tight, but the exported material doesn't always have to tell you everything. Be wise about where you get your water from. Alkaline water is best for your body.

Your body holds on to waste unless you drink water, which removes old stale water and replaces it with new water.

Waste water can also cause weight gain in your midsection. Like I said, be wise and smart about what you put in your body.

Don't eat or drink to the point where you feel bloated or very full. When you start to feel full stop drinking and eating.

Chapter 9 ~ Carbs/Fats/Protein

Protein:

I've heard it all the time. "I need more protein, protein, protein." You do need protein but you should be eating the right type of protein, which is lean protein.

Things like veggies have a little bit of protein in them. Try to have a smoothie with protein powder and add protein based foods.

Here are some protein containing foods that you can use for a snack or as a meal during the day: peanuts, almonds, pecans, natural peanut butter on whole grain toast, oatmeal, a turkey sandwich, chicken salad, tofu, lean ground beef, beans, tempeh, fish, and salmon.

These are just a few protein ideas you can try in order to get more protein into your nutrition plan and help you achieve your goals faster.

Today you need to understand the basics of protein and what it does for your body. When you are working out, you are ripping muscle fibres.

It's when you are resting and eating protein after your workout that rebuilding processes start making your muscles bigger and stronger.

Your eating plan and your specific goals determine how much protein you need to consume. You should eat at least 40% protein at every meal.

If you're a man, then your portion of meat protein should be at least as big as your fist. For a woman it should be half a fist.

A half fist should be the portion of protein per meal, but not the entire day. Three fist amounts should be your total amount of meat per day for men and 1.5 fists for women.

That is the main calculation used in many weight loss programs. It is also helpful if you want to maintain your weight.

Always look at the nutrition facts of a food to see how much protein it contains. Keep your eye on the facts, and count how much protein is in each serving size, not the entire box.

Getting the body you want will take time. It involves math, mental strength and breaking emotional barriers. Protein is a big help. It repairs muscle soreness quickly.

Protein is one of the most important parts of rebuilding the muscle tissue in your body.

Carbs:

Definition: carbs are a fuel source to give you energy to perform any activities, throughout the day. Remember when your mom asked you to eat your veggies?

She was trying to get you to eat the healthy natural foods that your body needs. If you say, "I don't like plain veggies," then try to spice them up and make a veggie stir fry with some flavor.

Next time you have a smoothie, add some kale or spinach, and I guarantee that you will not taste the veggies in your smoothie.

You're getting your daily veggies in, without even thinking about it. We also need to remember that carbohydrates are a fuel source, not a pleasure food.

Carbs give you energy and give you the fuel you need for your workout. Simple Carbs are fruits and grains; complex carbs are veggies.

I would recommend that you eat simple carbs for breakfast and lunch, then eat the complex carbs for lunch and dinner.

Stay away from breads in the evening. It is good to eat more veggies and meat at dinner. Starchy carbs are white rice, breads, and pastas.

Starchy carbs are full of sugars and are not healthy for you because white flour turns into sugar during digestion.

Eat more simple carbohydrates which are whole wheat grains and cereals which have all the nutrients, minerals and vitamins the body needs.

You want to have at least 30% carbohydrates in your nutrition plan.

Fats:

We hear it all the time that fats are bad for you and you should avoid them at all costs, which is not entirely true.

There are some good fats out there, in fact, if we didn't have any fats in our diet we would probably get sick. There are a few fats you should add into your meals.

For example: coconut oil, flax seeds, chia seeds and avocado. These foods contain a few healthy and natural fats that you can put into your meals.

Whether it's a salad or a spice on our lean meats, be creative with your food, because there are millions of ways to make a meal. You can mix and match spices instead of using salt and pepper for everything.

Here are the most common types of fats: saturated fat, trans-fat, monounsaturated fat and polyunsaturated fat.

Be careful of saturated fats because they will increase your blood pressure and cholesterol. Saturated fat is commonly found in fast food.

Polyunsaturated and monounsaturated fats are high in omega 3 and 6 which are things we want in our body. Omega 3 and 6 help reduce the chance of getting heart disease or high blood pressure.

The good fats to look for are fish oils, seafood, Brazil nuts, walnuts, and seeds. Stay away from whole milk, baked goods such as biscuits, pastries, fatty meats and fried fast food.

Learn what to look for and what to avoid so that you can make clean eating a lifestyle. Eat clean and healthy fats. In the recipe section you will see some of the healthy fats, carbs and proteins.

Chapter 10 ~ Exercise Program

FITNESS:

So you've heard people talking about fitness and how good it is for you. It's time to get started!

Ultimately, fitness doesn't have to be about workouts in the gym, it can be doing sports or doing activities with your family or friends or just going for a nice walk. This is what I think fitness means:

F is for Focus,

I is for Interest,

T is for Trust,

N is for Nutrition,

E is for Education,

S is for Strength

S is for Spirit.

Find the inner self to help you to keep going and focus on yourself and your fitness goals. I am going to demonstrate all these exercises and show you the proper form for them.

Use a program to lose weight, lose fat, burn calories, and gain muscle mass. Fitness is so much more than the outward appearance.

It's about feeling better about yourself and touching base with your spirit and emotions. Fitness is about learning about yourself and how to be a better person.

We as a culture are so narrow minded about fitness. We need to broaden our thinking towards it. I will explain every portion of this program and get you started on your way to becoming the person you were created to be.

Let's get started. There will be millions of sceptics that will judge without trying what you will try. Getting started is the first step toward getting the body and life you were made for.

Exercise Types:

Intentional exercise is going to change the path on how you feel about yourself and look at yourself in the mirror. I will show you how to take your body to peak physical condition.

This program will be hard, but nothing worthwhile in life is easy. That is why I am here to help you on your way and guide you in the right direction.

Cardio:

Let's talk about the cardio portion of the program. Cardio improves the heart and prevents heart attacks. The cardio portion of this program ranges from beginner to advanced exercises.

I will include a cardio exercise plan in this book that will help you achieve different goals from burning fat to losing weight.

I love it when people understand that six pack abs do not come from crunches, but instead they come from doing cardio exercise. Once you burn the fat off your midsection you will see the abs underneath.

There are a few different types of cardio for different skill levels. The first steps are walking, running and jogging.

This program is going to start small with these exercises. In the beginning you don't have to worry about getting too advanced and getting stressed about not knowing how to do the exercises.

The three beginner workouts will be easy and will not require too much brain work. I'll tell you what to do and how to do it, all you have to do is follow the instructions and go for it and do your best.

The second component is body resistance exercises including plyometrics and sports drills that will help you train like an expert and take your body to the next level of fitness without using any machines or equipment.

This leap will challenge, but looking well and getting healthy will come with hard work. There is going to be a cardio section that is designed to help improve your cardiovascular fitness and improve your breath control and blood pressure.

Strength:

I am going to show you resistance training with just your body. This way, you don't have to spend money on gym memberships and you can work out in private.

I understand that you probably don't like people staring at you in the gym because it can get overwhelming, especially when starting out. Start small and work your way up.

Don't listen to the comments some people say about you; I don't care what they think. I care about who you say you are.

You are valued and worth getting in the best shape of your life. Ignore the negative comments that you have heard, they don't matter.

Remember, strength isn't just physical it includes physiological strength. It's not easy but it will be worth it.

Bodily resistance training is about starting with the basics and then working your way up. Don't feel pressured or overwhelmed by this program, simply go at your own pace.

Remember, this is a lifestyle and there is no finish line. Take your time, because you have the rest of your life to achieve your goals.

In strength training it is important to think about how to maneuver your own body weight and control your body properly.

Form is more important to me than just getting big muscles. Honestly, some people who have big muscles sometimes struggle with bodyweight exercise because they are not used to it.

We all need to be aware that we live in this body and need to learn how to work with it. Next up, we will learn about lower body and upper body training to show different variation and modification for different fitness levels. Always work at your own range of motion and flexibility.

Strength with Dumbbells:

I will show you how training with dumbbells can be effective and beneficial for you and can even be fun and give you a smile. We will be exercising the upper and lower body together and separate for two reasons.

The first reason to do them together is that you burn more calories when you exercise just your upper body or just your lower body.

Working both together while using your core helps you burn fat faster. Your legs are the largest muscle group in your body. So when you add upper body into the exercise it becomes even better.

Two reasons to work the upper and lower body separate is to attack a certain muscle and sculpt it so it can bulk and become more pronounced.

I want you to see people and show them what you can do with strength and disprove the myth about strength training.

Lifting 10lbs weight won't get you huge or bulky. Ladies and gentlemen, don't be afraid to lift weights. It can even lean you out more if you add weights. Be proud of what you have done.

Free weights are especially beneficial if you have proper form. If your form is bad you have a high chance of hurting yourself.

Yoga:

Yoga is the fountain of youth. I am going to show you how holding isometric poses can help you to reduce your stress levels and calm the body, mind and soul.

Through doing slow fluent movements yoga can help lengthen muscles without putting stress on the body, as opposed to the hard pounding of cardio training.

I'm going to put you through a flow of flexibility and meditating poses to help calm you down and get an effective workout in without pressure on the joints.

Yoga defines how young you are by your spine. If your spine is not flexible you are old. If your spine is flexible you are young. Yoga is a way to relax and reduce anxiety, depression and sadness.

Yoga can help how you feel in your own skin, loving everything about who you are.

Abs/Core:

Training your mid-section is all about keeping yourself balanced and stabilized at work or doing your daily activities.

Your abs are very important. I would recommend you to do balance and core stability work which improves your posture and mobility.

The stronger your abs are the stronger your lower back will be in any position. When you stand tall, the strength is coming from your midsection to help with your posture, balance and form.

I recommend to do core work at any age and any level. Core exercise is something you can do for the rest of your life.

Try Pilates for an abs, butt and thigh workout, it will help reduce pain if you have it. I will help you along this process to get you to where you want to go.

Your core stability the most important aspect of fitness. Your abs will be put through a program to get them stronger and more flexible than before.

Chapter 11 ~ God's View of Fitness

I want to tell why God is part of your fitness process and how the spiritual side can be a part of your health.

You would be surprised how many verses in the bible talk about fitness. Words like strength, health, and power are all in the bible.

We need to know that we all have a soul and we need to take care of the soul and nurture it with care and love just the like we care for our body.

1 Corinthians 6:19-20 - 19 or do you not know that your body is a temple of the Holy Spirit within you, whom you have from God? You are not your own, 20 for you were bought with a price. So glorify God in your body.

1 Corinthians 3:17-17 if anyone destroys God's temple, God will destroy him. For God's temple is holy, and you are that temple.

1 Timothy 4:8-8 for while bodily training is of some value, godliness is of value in every way, as it holds promise for the present life and also for the life to come.

1 Corinthians 9:24-27-24 Do you not know that in a race all the runners run, but only one receives the prize? So run that you may obtain it. 25 Every athlete exercises self-control in all things. They do it to receive a perishable wreath, but we are imperishable. 26 So I do not run aimlessly; I do not box as one beating the air. 27 But I discipline my body and keep it under control, lest after preaching to others I myself should be disqualified.

1 Corinthians 3:16-16 Do you not know that you[a] are God's temple and that God's Spirit dwells in you?

1 Corinthians 10:31-31 so whether you eat or drink, or whatever you do, do all to the glory of God.

Isaiah 40:31-but they who wait for the LORD shall renew their strength;

    They shall mount up with wings like eagles;

They shall run and not be weary;

    They shall walk and not faint.

Proverbs 31:17-She dresses herself with strength

    And makes her arms strong.

What all these verses have in common is that they talk about fitness. My approach to fitness isn't just physical.

It's more about the inward appearance and how you feel and deal with your emotional and mental side, how to release all negative thoughts and emotions that are inside and get them out of your system.

I want to tell you how this changes the way you look at fitness and God. I believe that God created fitness to be a tool to change lives and show people God's love through fitness.

I want to show people how we can be happy and love what we have been given and value it. Our bodies are built to help and repair themselves.

All this damage we do to our bodies stops the fluid movement of blood, or the contraction of the active muscle fibres.

I believe God has a purpose for our bodies, he created them for a reason. We were meant to work and meant to keep everything flowing properly and safely.

1 timothy 4:8 talks about how physical training is valuable. This book was written about 2,000 years ago!

If it talks about modern culture and modern activates, this tells me that God values what he created and wants us to take care of his creation.

It's like if you ask a friend to take care of your flowers and then after a week he forgot to water them and destroyed the flowers.

We sometimes forget or don't care if we don't follow through with the task that is given to us. We say we will do it but don't always follow through.

Imagine how God feels when we are lazy and don't care if we become big and let our weight get out of control. God lives inside of us and when we don't love or treasure our bodies enough and destroy what he gave to us, it's like a slap in the face.

We say, I think I know better than the big man upstairs and I know how to care for my body. In *1 Corinthians 9: 24-27* it talks about running the race.

Let's pause there for a second. What does that mean to you? What race are we running? Think about it. Is it a physical or spiritual battle, or it is an emotional and mental battle in our life?

It's how we learn to deal with the challenges of the race of life. Do you run away from problems or dive in head first?

I believe once you understand what your race is, learn to deal with those unexpected situations, before you know it you have created the life you always wanted to live.

The next point I want to say is that every athlete exercises self-control in one way or another. How is self-control and running a race part of this topic of what God thinks about fitness?

Think before you judge or say a smart comment about this. What are you feeling right now about God or fitness? Maybe you think it's all not true.

Let me ask you this, how would people in the bible know that fitness or physical training is valued, even 2000 years ago?

Be slow to speak and quick to listen, take note of this and make sure you remember what I'm saying. If you think I'm wrong, prove to me that God doesn't value our bodies and lives.

God designed our bodies with endorphins that get released when we workout which make us feel happy about ourselves. God knew this would help people change the path of their lives.

There are no loopholes weight loss or toning up. It's hard work getting in the gym to feel better about ourselves and getting the life and body you always wanted.

God gave us fruits since the beginning, and God knew the power of nutrition and physical and spiritual training.

I think just as Hollywood knows how to use that spiritual power and world more than anyone else, but it's not from God, it's from Satan.

Demonic power is as real as God's power. My point is that God loves you so much that he wants you to get as much out of your life as possible.

The only way you can do that is to take care of your life and body. Your body is a gift from God and no one needs to destroy it for selfish pleasure. Everyone, including ourselves, needs to treasure what is given to us.

Chapter 12 ~ Food Journal

Let's talk about the benefits of having a food journal. When it comes to losing inches or weight it comes down to one thing, portion control. You are probably asking why I need to keep a food journal.

Let me ask you, do you have a personal journal? Write down all you have done. Do you need a record of your life on paper? Do you need to keep track of how you feel?

It's important to go back and look over the journal and see proven results. Say you got in a car accident, do you keep record of the licence plate and get their information to make sure everyone is safe and okay?

When it comes to weight loss it's important to keep a record of your progress, to know how far you have come. Track how many calories you eat each meal and write it down.

A food journal is more than just writing down what you're eating, it's a change of heart on how you will feel. It's gaining the knowledge of why you look the way you do.

I'm trying to express to you that there is proof in the effort you put. I want you to trust me that I know what I'm talking about when it comes to gaining control over your life.

A food journal is something to give you a helping hand to get started on your toning or weight loss goals. Once you know how many calories are in your foods it all changes.

A journal is a tool I recommend to use when you first get started on your fitness goals. You can stick with it for as long as you want, but if you're just starting I would give you two options.

First you can keep on journaling once you know how much a teaspoon or cup is, then you will be able to recognize how much food is in a serving.

The second option is you can keep going with the food journal to keep you on the right track and won't slip up, let's be honest, we all slip up from time to time.

These guidelines are tools that you can use for reality and make sure you get success. My choice would be to stick with the food journal all the way, because the point of a food journal is to learn how to count calories.

Because in Canada we don't know what a serving size is anymore train your eye and brain to know how much a serving size is.

Most fast food places will give a plate of food and will call it one serving, in reality it is probably two or three servings. We usually don't want to do the calculation because math is hard.

You probably do a lot of math at work for a sort of reasons, to build up the company or to produce more product. You might not like it, but it gets you food and shelter.

Doing math for health should be just as motivating. Did you know that in the long run, eating fast food is more expensive than eating healthy meals at home?

You keep track of your bills and money, why not keep track of your food intake because it will help you to feel so much better in the long hall.

Life is tough, but we do things so we can be successful. I work my butt off to make sure I know what I can afford and spend as little as possible.

A food journal is going to be a lifestyle, not a short term gimmick. You can do it short term, but I bet if you keep at it for the long run you will feel more relief, support and encouragement knowing you accomplished something.

Chapter 13 ~ Drinking and Smoking

This part is all about smoking and drinking. We are going to start with smoking. Here's a question, why do we smoke? What benefit does it have to our bodies?

Is it because it gives you a high which makes you feel happy. I am going to give you an illustration to help you understand what I will be talking about.

First, think of your heart, it's pumping blood to your body, then image that you were a kid till now and you have a small black circle in the middle of your heart.

That small black circle is called a void in our life. We don't know how to cope with stress or pressure. So we temporarily deal with our problems.

As humans we have needs and we feel the need to fill that black circle in our heart with anything that will make us feel satisfied.

We smoke with the cool guys and for that short time the black hole will go away. Once you are finished partying, the void will come back. Once we need this temporary fix all the time, it becomes an addiction.

When you breathe smoke into your lungs it damages the cells that help pump blood and oxygen to the muscles.

Let me ask you, what is the point of fire? Fire is created to burn material into small molecules and turn it into ash. Is the fire of a cigarette benefiting your body or destroying it?

Sometimes you feel pain or cramping because the smoke is slowing down life processes. When you are smoking you tend to cough because something is entering your system that is not wanted.

It's an extra we put into our body that destroys our liver, lungs, heart and brain. Smoke burns up brain cells and will make you go crazy and do stuff you would never dream of.

The human body is so complex that we need to do everything we can to keep it moving, functioning and growing.

This is where your life will change and be flipped completely around. You will see that you don't need this smoking habit.

Once you look at the science behind how bad smoking is, it will surprise you even as a smoker. I don't want to put you down if you are a smoker, but I want to help you understand what you're getting into.

It only takes one step before you will slip into temptation and damage your body and your friendships. Be smart and wise about how you will take your next step.

Next, I want to tell you there is hope on the other side. I want to do any and everything I can to help you reach your goal and overcome any obstacles that are in the way.

The first step is recognizing you have a smoking problem.

The second step is to reduce the amount of cigarettes you smoke per day.

The third step is to get people in your life that will lift you up. Get a support group to help you and ask you every day if you smoked.

The fourth step is to go to a counsellor to tell you what to substitute a cigarette for and find true satisfaction.

The fifth step is to quit once and for all. Never let yourself fall back into the bad habit. Keep your eyes open and ready and take these steps that will help you change the pattern of your life forever.

Sometimes tough love hurts and I'm here to tell you to man up and start taking care of what was given to you and stop wasting it and pretending it's useless.

I can't tell you about your health, I want to be that light in your life that will shine through. I am going to do what it takes to be your teacher and guide you into the direction you need to go. I will never give up hope. Start small and work your way up.

Chapter 14 ~ Body Obsession

Body obsession is a big deal in this world and culture. There are plenty of people becoming models and showing off their body, bodybuilders caring about the huge ripped muscles and how they look amazing, bikini models showing off their toned and tightened flat abs and lean legs and arms.

We need to learn not to obsess about how we look all the time. A lot of people in the fitness industry dwell on the physical appearance, thinking that physical appearance is what life is all about.

Some people care too much about what other people think about their looks and their performance at the beach or gym.

When it comes to fitness a lot of bodybuilders and yoga people care about how their muscles look on the outside. We often let how we look play a big part in our life and we let it change how we act towards others.

Before we know it, our body becomes more important than anything else; our work, family, friends, and God have come second to our body.

We spend money on protein powder, gainer, and pre workout. We show off our bodies and tell others how much we lift and how our muscles look so visible and sculpted for perfection.

It's not healthy to be obsessed over anything, especially our bodies. There is more to life than just thinking about how we look and act.

Human's emotions are more important and dealing with the inner self can help you to avoid worshiping your own body.

I want to make a point right here to say that there are four aspects to fitness: emotional, mental, spiritual and physical.

If you focus on just your physical appearance, it becomes a body obsession. How do I look? Are my biceps better, my abs more ripped?

Why don't we seem to care about the other aspects of fitness? In reality, there are people who go to the gym because they hate the way they look and want to change it without changing their mindset or dealing with emotional baggage.

Body obsession is not healthy if you don't touch on the inner self and deal with problems that may make you go to the gym for the wrong reasons. It's all about how we approach the situation.

Don't look at your body in the mirror without saying to yourself, I changed the route of my life from the inside out.

Chapter 15 ~ Treat Day/Cheat Day

So I want to talk about cheat day/treat day. It has to be one of the most important aspects of the fitness and nutrition industry.

We all have the question, when can I enjoy a pizza or ice cream? This is an important aspect to know. Every trainer and person will give you a different answer.

I want to help you understand my view of splurging and treating yourself in the proper manner and amount.

When you are on my nutrition plan and do it for at least four weeks, you can enjoy junk food while staying on a good healthy eating plan.

First, if you want to lose weight, we all get on the same page so we can get this plan started. The first thing I will say is, everything in moderation.

That doesn't mean you stuff your face full of broccoli and then say I can eat a cookie because I ate healthy, it doesn't work that way. We need to learn the moderation method.

I want you to know how to enjoy a splurge meal in a weight loss or toning setting. We all feel we deserve to earn some treats after a long hard day at work.

Why do we put good tasting foods under the bus? We can enjoy great tasting healthy meals without thinking it's healthy. Cheat days are okay in my books or this book.

What I will say is I will give you a cheat guide to follow. Remember it's a lifestyle not a permanent fix, in the first month you will have no cheat day. You say WHAT?!

Listen, what I need to do is go through a cleansing period before you can start to treat yourself. The reason for that is our taste buds are so saturated from canned foods and fast food so we need to learn to not rely on saturated and processed foods.

Our tongue, mouth and eyes don't understand what is good and what is bad anymore. We need to help our eyes, mouth, and tongue to know what a proper serving size looks like.

On top of that, we need to transform the way we taste and eat food because as you eat healthier your taste buds will change. I will have a bunch of new tasty and healthy meals for you to choose from to help you on your way to success. In the second month we will start cheat days.

Here is the plan: There's 7 days a week, I made a chart to follow, I want you to enjoy the foods you like in moderation.

Week 1: 6 day clean meals 1 cheat day.

Monday: Clean Meal

Tuesday: Clean Meal

Wednesday: Clean Meal

Thursday: Clean Meal

Friday: Cheat Day

Saturday: Clean Meal

Sunday: Clean Meal

Week 2: 5 days clean eating 2 cheats days

Monday: Clean Meal

Tuesday: Clean Meal

Wednesday: Cheat Day

Thursday: Clean Meal

Friday: Clean Meal

Saturday: Clean Meal

Sunday: Cheat Day

Week 3: 6 clean meals 1 cheat day

Monday: Clean Meal

Tuesday: Clean Meal

Wednesday: Clean Meal

Thursday: Cheat Day

Friday: Clean Meal

Saturday: Clean Meal

Sunday: Clean Meal

Week 4: 5 healthy meals 2 cheat days.

Monday: Clean Meal

Tuesday: Clean Meal

Wednesday: Clean Meal

Thursday: Cheat Day

Friday: Clean Meal

Saturday: Clean Meal

Sunday: Cheat Day

I will give you some options that will lower the calories for your cheat days and still allow you to enjoy a guilt-free dessert without the extra calories.

For example: Low fat ice cream with M&Ms, a small chocolate cake, a hot dog on a whole wheat bun with mustard and a bowl of chips.

These are just a few ideas that we can learn from and teach ourselves and our peers to become healthier and cleaner on the inside and feel so much better after, because we can enjoy life because we are human.

We all need to have some tips for snacks we can try: a glass of wine is okay once in a while, Organic black coffee, a small piece of a chocolate bar, small sized popcorn and even some Reese cups.

Chapter 16 ~ Judgment/Attitude

Let's start talking about your approach to fitness. first of all, I want you to tell me the first few things that come to your mind when I say (Fitness)

_____
_____
_____
_____
_____
_____

So why do you think that certain way about fitness?

Is it because someone told you this is what it is, or you made it up from your own view or opinion on it. What's the reason behind all your thinking?

We judge too quickly in our culture and need to get our facts straight before we start saying something we might regret. It's like the old phrase goes, don't judge a book by its cover. You need to get inside an issue and read about it before you can make the call on what you think of it.

Don't just skip through a topic and say you hate it when you just scanned the topic. You need to get out of the quick mindset of judgment. Learn about what you are talking about before you judge it.

Attitude and judgement go hand in hand in life. How is your attitude toward fitness or health in general? If you're like, I don't need fitness, it's stupid.

Then I think you need to think about what you say before you say it. Get well educated about why your health is important in the first place.

If you have had a bad attitude, we need to help untwist the thoughts that cause it. I think fitness can help improve our attitudes.

Fitness is the capability of the body to distribute inhaled oxygen to muscle tissue during increased physical effort.

Why judge if you don't even know the root cause or why it was created in the first place. Listen to me, when I tell you something new or a fact on fitness I want you to go search it up because I want you to have the knowledge to know the different parts of fitness and the benefits they have for you.

I can't say, I hate trampolines, if I have never been on one. You need to try something before you make assumptions.

I want to question your attitude and judgement for a second. Why do you act and talk a certain way about a certain object or action that you haven't taken part of yet?

What is your reason behind that? I care about your attitude and the thoughts of judgment right now. Put fitness to the side for now let's talk about attitude – this is for you personally to write down.

Describe your personality on the space below:

_____
_____
_____
_____
_____
_____

So let's talk about this attitude how it affects how you talk.

I'm going to be your fitness counsellor for the moment. Do you have a grudge toward someone? Has someone bullied you? Have you been abused? What is the root of your anger and bitterness?

Our attitude shows through actions. When I see someone's attitude toward you, I know that they have been tampered with themselves and people twisted their emotions and thoughts toward something they loved.

The love they had is gone and the only satisfaction they feel is from judging someone for what used to be love. I will talk about pain and hurts in the next chapter, but in this chapter I want to change a negative attitude and show more options and patterns for your life.

This judgment and attitude change process will take time and effort. Before you judge someone or something, ask yourself one question: why? Find the root cause.

This is really deep stuff, but sometimes people don't want to talk about their issues or problems but if you don't talk about it all of your situations will be bottled up inside and destroy you.

I am doing this because I care about your wellness as much as your health. They go hand in hand. We need to discuss this to break through physical and emotional barriers and go on to the other side seeing success and fulfillment.

After this talk I hope that the depressing part is done. I want to shine the light on the darkness and show you the way out of this situation.

The first step is telling someone your problems and not bottle it up inside, the second step is to find a mentor and get them to encourage you and to keep you on the right track and go for coffee.

Third, take time to meditate on all the positive accomplishments you have done in your life, or by saying positive words from small to big things.

For example: I am beautiful, valued, I helped my brother with their homework, I drove someone to school, I fed the homeless, I love myself and others. These are a few examples of positive accomplishments you have done and special things about you.

I believe in you and I know you can do all things when you set your mind to it. Believe in yourself and the power of the mental strength you can do in this world.

Changing the world's attitude towards people by being a light and not looking down upon people. Refuse to judge people and the world will take notice.

We all have problems and we all need support that is why we can work better as a team than as an individual.

Today's culture is judging of people. It tells us that we need to look the look and act the part to fit in. We need to learn that we have different ways to react and communicate when we deal with situations.

For example: If I think about a stranger or friend at school we may think "man, this guy has an attitude." That is not how we should act around others.

When someone judges too quickly and starts thinking negatively about how someone treats them, their judging becomes obvious and they say what's on their mind.

We need to understand that a lot of people have opinions of who you are and how you act in public. We can't let this get the best of us and we need to focus on how we can flip it around and turn it upside down when it is not what we want it to be.

This will turn the situation completely around, it will show you how you are progressing through these weeks and months, taking a look back on the first day till now and seeing how your attitude has changed.

Through these exercises you will become alerted of your old and new attitude. When negative or positive comments come up we learn to talk and say the right words instead of saying everything that's on our mind about what just happened. I deeply care about your physical health as much as your mental and emotional health.

What I want you to do is write down how you really feel. Why you are the way you are and why you are where you are at now with your weight, etc.

_____
_____
_____
_____
_____
_____

Chapter 17 ~ Pain And Hurts

We are going to talk about pain and hurts. The emotional side of how we have been hurt and the pains we carry around.

We are going to talk about the pains of others that get carried over and the hurts from an injury. These are the three main topics we will be talking about this segment.

First is the emotional hurts and pains. We need to get deep into the roots and see what the big picture is here.

Why are we hurting and having this pain?

_____

What is the root cause of all this?

_____

I want to start getting you thinking about what I can do as your trainer/mentor to overcome hurdles and get you away from your past. I want to mentor you.

Today we are talking about how to deal with emotional baggage. You've heard when you were a kid that sticks and stones may break your bones but words will never hurt me.

That is a lie we teach our kids, even in our school we teach them that it's okay. Words are powerful and have a huge part in your mental and emotional reaction towards particular life situations.

We need to use the right tools to be uplifting to others and strengthen them with encouraging words and give them the right tools to deal with this problem area.

First, when you have emotional hurt and pain we need to learn how to control the trigger of emotions.

Talk about your hurts and pains, don't hold it in because that will be damaging to you and will eat you up inside and kill your positive side.

People hurt others to lift themselves up and be proud of what they have done. Ask someone to mentor you and guide you in the right direction and learn how to react in the right way next time it happens.

Don't always react negatively because we are born imperfect and we tend to lean on the negative/harmful side. Be the optimistic one who lives in the opposite spirit.

It's going to be a process to deal with this emotion. Because emotional people are sensitive, they need their hearts to be loved on.

As your fitness counsellor I love you and want to make a difference in how you view yourself when you look in the mirror or look around you.

You were created on purpose and for a purpose, you are not a mistake and you were placed on this earth for a reason. Don't let your pain get the best of you.

The second point I want to look at is root causes. When you see a tree with beautiful fruits and leaves, nice bark, trunk in good soil, it is there because of this one thing: THE ROOTS.

Emotional pain cuts deep inside and we don't always deal with it in the right way. Why are you cutting your body to cure the deep emotional problems? How does physical pain and suffering help the inner healing? How does it fix all the spiritual, mental and emotional heartache?

Let's talk just about pain right now. It's about to get real. Put fitness on the side for now. We are going to talk about painful thoughts.

Right now it's about the pain and hurts that people have done in our lives and have crushed our hopes and dreams. It's going to be hard to read this, but it needs to get said, so bear with me.

But remember, I'm writing this so that you can overcome the pain and enjoy your life. I'm going to tell a story to give you some perspective.

Think back to when you were a little kid, how you felt at school and how your peers treated you. Did they push you around and bully you? Did they abuse you or did you get into a fight? As you grew up, what caused you to do what you do now?

People tell me sad stories; that they cut themselves because their ex sexually abused them. Why are you so depressed I ask?

Some people have never felt loved and everyone that they come in contact with hates on them and tells them they're dumb, stupid, ugly and worthless.

They now find no value in themselves and think that they are not worth saving or putting any time into. Some people have drinking problems because of the pain, and want me to just pretend it never happened.

Please stop and leave this addiction. They tell me they can't, it's a part of who they are, that their father was drunk in front of them when they were a kid and he would hurt them so much that they grew up into this, it's a family chain.

They feel that no one could want to respect them for who they are. Their father physically and verbally abused them when they were children and they have been scared to talk and connect with him because he always talks negative to them.

We cry out, why, why, why does this happen to me? What did I do wrong? I want just one person to say I LOVE YOU and think I am worth more than dirt. Let me pause there for a second. Why am I talking about this?

I think we need to know that people in this world are dying from depression, abuse and hatred from other horrible situations. They commit suicide and believe there is no other exit out. For all these people I want to share a word with you from the Bible:

John 16:33: "I have told you these things, so that in me you may have peace. In this world you will have trouble. But take heart! I have overcome the world".

2 Corinthians 1:3-4: "Praise be to the God and Father of our Lord Jesus Christ, the Father of compassion and the God of all comfort, who comforts us in all our troubles, so that we can comfort those in any trouble with the comfort we ourselves receive from God".

I know that when I sink my teeth into the problem I will get the solution and get to where I need to be and get help to get rid of any pain or hurts from the past.

What I described to you is situations people have been through in this world. We need to know that we can fight for them and show them that there is more to life then what is happening now to them.

In the next chapter we will talk about forgiveness, but I want you to help yourself know why we go through hard painful hurts in our life.

If we would go through life and not experience any pain, struggles or problems how do you think this world would be today?

It would be completely different or even flipped around and your brains would function differently. We have all heard the phrase, when you fall down you pick yourself back up. It's important.

Don't let past hurts or pain define you for who you are today. I believe we go through struggles so that we learn from past mistakes and overcome problems in our life and learn to not repeat them.

During hurts and pains that are very harsh, it is very hard to understand that there is going to be a light at the end of the tunnel; it's going to be okay. Life is going to get better, but life will always have struggles.

The more we wrap our brains around the fact that there are struggles, the more we will move on from what did happen and prepare for what is going to happen next in story of my life.

The point of the story is that pains help us break through unwanted walls to get to where we want to be in life. Though, getting to where you want comes with challenges.

Success only comes when you fail, true successful people failed and then work towards their realistic goal of the imaged life.

I want you to image this and see where I'm going with it. Let's say you're on a long straight road and every time you get hurt you land in a puddle. The puddle represents our problems.

There are many puddles on this straight path, but when you build a bridge over top you are overcoming your problems and solving them.

Then you look back and say, hey, I built myself up and overcame some hurdles in life. Then comes another puddle you trip and fall down but learn from the last puddle that you overcame that problem and move forward.

Now you are aware of these puddles and can learn to work around them and overcome them. This is not the end as there will be more puddles, but I know and believe that you will overcome and get through it and learn from your past mistakes and learn how to not fall as often.

Learn to stand firm on the foundation of success. Focus on the positive and loving people who care about you.

Now we are starting to get rid of grief and pains from our past or present life. Here are a few steps to help you out.

1 Step: Acknowledge you need help.

2 Step: Tell someone close to you what you are or did deal with in your life. Telling someone is the first step and helps you to get rid of some pain. It tells me you are truly ready to get out of this rut.

3 Step: Get group support or a counsellor to help you through this.

4 Step: Invest in positive music and novels that bring light into your life.

5 Step: Meditate and pray

6 Step: Get on this fitness and nutrition plan to kick-start your success. When you try brutal and hard exercise movements, unwanted emotions raise to the surface, instead of yelling at someone; possibly hitting a friend or spouse.

You express yourself through certain movements. With my coaching I'll guide you through the tough times, we are in this journey together. The road to succeed is not easy, but nothing's easy in life anyway.

Chapter 18 ~ Forgive Yourself And Forgive Others

Fitness has more than one aspect or goal. In this segment we are going to be talking about forgiveness. This segment is so important when it comes to your lifestyle and your wellness goals.

Sometimes we overlook our past problems that can have an effect on our workouts. We need to learn to let go of our past and get rid of negative power that we hang on to.

If it is bitterness in your life towards a certain group, friends, family, work, or public situation, we need to get rid of it before it takes over our lives. Bitterness eats us up inside.

I know I am human and I deal with bitterness to people who have hurt me deeply, but I'm learning that it's a process to forgive someone, it doesn't happen overnight, it takes time.

Same goes for you, you need to learn to get work through situations in the right way. I am going to give you a formula to help get you started on forgiving others and yourself.

I want you to write down on the lines below who you have bitterness towards. Once you write that down I want you to ask yourself, why do I dwell on this and what benefit does it have for me?

Then, I want you to pray and say I am sorry for all the hatred I had toward this company or person. I forgive these people for what they did to me.

You don't need to think about whether they will forgive you back or not, that's their problems not yours. Your job is to do your part and go up to that person or write a letter saying that you forgive them for all the damage they did to you.

Now, write it down and with all your heart say I am sorry and I forgive you.

_____
_____
_____
_____
_____
_____
_____
_____
_____
_____

After you forgive them whole heartedly with all your heart, soul and mind you will start to slowly feel better about yourself.

Like I said, letting go of all the bitterness, hatred or anger toward a certain group or person will take time, but once you commit and make that decision to want to feel better towards these people and yourself, you will not want to live in regret anymore.

Next, I want to say that beating ourselves up is something we need to target, we should learn that we are as valued as anyone else. No matter the background or what they have done. We tend to beat ourselves up for the smallest things.

For example, I embarrassed myself in front of the class during my speech. When this happens we say in our head that we failed, stumbled on that word, I'm stupid.

In school class projects, why do we get worked up and over and over let our small problems get the best of us? Then we will dwell on that for the rest of the day.

In reality, I don't care about that small incident in class. Guess what? It's going to happen again. How will you react when it happens again?

Do we beat ourselves up and say, it's hopeless, or do we say, I fell down, but I will get back up and not let my past define who I am today? I sometimes think we dwell on the past mistakes too much.

Here's another tip: forgive and forget. It's that simple. It's an easy term, but it's not easy to do. It takes time to process and choose to forget what you already did.

Why bother trying so hard to remember what you did and focus on that pain? When we focus on the past pain it reflects on how we live our life today.

I want to give you an example: I'm going to tell you a bit of a story. Back in the day there was a kid who had problems with communication and struggled to speak English.

He got picked on because he had a learning disability and people told him that he wouldn't be successful in his dream of art.

This kid refused to listen to his peers and quit school and followed his passion and heart for becoming an artist. Let me tell you something.

If that kid would've listened to his classmates, then his life would have been different as we know it. Who was he? His name was Walt Disney, yes Walt Disney had a learning disability and he didn't let that stop him from doing what he loved.

There are celebrities and famous people who have these same problems. If they kept putting themselves down, and had never believed in themselves, then you would have never seen any Disney movies.

Don't let your past define you. Forgive and forget, forgive and forget, forgive and forget. It's that simple. I am here to support you. By the way, you can follow me on my social media where I give motivation that may help you face that fear.

Don't get me wrong it's going to be hard, but I believe in you. Get a support group and ask people who you can trust to keep you accountable and you will be able to succeed in your life goals.

I believe you can do it and when you feel bad about something you did or something someone did to you, say, I forgive them every day, even if it wasn't your fault.

Don't say it in a sassy voice, but in a sincere way. I forgive you. Say it from your heart and on an emotional level. Say, I am deeply so sorry for all the pain and suffering that happened and I forgive you and I forgive myself.

That's how you are going to face your emotional and mental feelings and forgive one another. I love this section of the chapter because it talks about the personal reality of emotions, bitterness, and negative thoughts.

Instead of beating yourself up with negative thoughts learn to manage them. We all need a close person to talk about life struggles, help get through the tough times.

This is one step closer to bettering yourself. To one degree or another we tend to not think about forgiveness all the time.

Why do you think that is? It could be because of our culture, peers, family, work, or friends. The list goes on and on.

I truly believe with all my heart that the deep cause of our problems comes from not forgiving and forgetting, and pretending an offence never happened without forgiving.

As time goes on we will feel upset and depressed and not know why. I guarantee that once we get to the roots of the tree, we will find out what that problem is and then learn how to deal with it in the right manner and cry out in your heart, saying I forgive myself for everything.

I FORGIVE EVERYONE who hurt me and I'm sorry for all my bad habits and behaviors, I want freedom. Once you get it out you will start to slowly feel better.

It takes time to get better and it needs to be a process that we work through every day. Say I forgive myself or others for what they have done to me.

Don't think it will be a quick fix or just a band aid or pretend it is all fine and perfect. It takes time to gain trust back and it takes time to forgive others and yourself.

Trust me, I struggle with this too, but I need to say I'm sorry and forgive all the broken things that have happened in my life from what I have done to myself or what others have done to me.

Trust the process and healing will happen and as time goes on it will change the path of your life. It will create new habits and patterns in how you approach others.

I believe you will overcome hurdles and obstacles, you will be the person you were meant to be, and live the life you were supposed to live.

This section was all about forgiveness and I believe you got a little freedom today by just forgiving.

Chapter 19 ~ Healthy Meal Plan/Recipes

Breakfast:

1 Serving Oatmeal

- 2/3 cup of water
- 1/3 cup of oatmeal
- 2 teaspoons natural peanut butter
- 2 teaspoons honey
- 1 cup of berry mix.

Oatmeal Pancakes 4 Servings

- ½ cup of whole wheat flour
- ½ cup of quick oatmeal
- 1 tablespoon of white sugar
- 1 teaspoon of baking powder
- ½ teaspoon of baking soda
- ¾ cup vanilla almond milk
- 1 teaspoon of vanilla extract
- 2 tablespoons of vegetable oil
- 1 egg

Oatmeal 1 Serving

- 1/3 cup of dry oats 2/3 cups water, dash of Salt

Directions:

- ✓ Put the 1/3 oats into a serving bowl,
- ✓ Add 2/3 cups of water,
- ✓ Microwave it for 2 minutes and it will be hot and ready to eat.

Fruit Bowl Salad 2 Servings

- 1 medium apple
- 1 cup of blueberries
- 1 teaspoon of cinnamon
- 2 teaspoons of agave
- Half a banana
- ½ cup blackberries

Directions:

- ✓ Get a serving bowl
- ✓ ½ cup of blackberries
- ✓ Dice the medium apple in the bowl
- ✓ Heat it up in microwave 30 seconds
- ✓ Add 1 teaspoon of cinnamon and agave
- ✓ Chop the half banana into small slices
- ✓ Ready to serve

English muffin

- Half English muffin
- 1 egg
- Dash of salt and pepper
- ½ teaspoon of chia Seeds
- ½ teaspoon of garlic
- ½ teaspoon of basil
- 2/3 cups Greek yogurt
- 1 teaspoon mustard seeds

Directions:

- ✓ Toast your English muffin in the toaster for about 1.5 minutes
- ✓ Put 1 egg in a small pan and heat at medium high
- ✓ Let it cook for 10 minutes
- ✓ Put a dash salt and pepper on the boiling egg
- ✓ In a separate bowl put ½ teaspoon chia seeds
- ✓ ½ teaspoon garlic
- ✓ ½ teaspoon basil
- ✓ 2/3 Greek yogurt or plain, microwave 1 minute

- ✓ Put the half English muffin on the plate then put the egg on top, for the dressing add the Greek yogurt and dressing for a healthy natural taste without adding extra calories.
- ✓ Now time to enjoy

Lunch Menu:
Salmon Salad

- 1 medium salmon
- 2 cups of kale
- 1 boiled egg
- 2 tablespoons Greek yogurt or plain yogurt
- 1 tablespoon hummus
- 1 cup of peppers, red, green, or yellow
- 1 cup of tomatoes

Directions:

- ✓ Put it in the oven at 400F for 25 minutes
- ✓ Chop up 1 pepper into small pieces
- ✓ Dice 1 tomato
- ✓ Chop the egg into thin strips put into another bowl
- ✓ Get another serving bowl for the dressing. Add 1 tablespoon of hummus and 2 tablespoons of Greek yogurt
- ✓ Chop up the kale finely and put it on the plate after you rinse the vegetable
- ✓ Put the salmon on after it has been cooked through all the way

BraydonsFitness.com

- Put the chopped and sliced peppers and tomatoes on, then after you stir the dressing, put it on top of the salad and enjoy.

Vegetarian Chilli 4 serving

- 1 cup tomato sauce
- 2/3 cups olive oil mayonnaise
- 2/3 cup organic BBQ sauce
- 1 whole tomato
- 1 cup of kale
- 1 cup of spinach
- 2/3 cup snow peas
- 1/3 cup red peppers
- 1/3 cup celery
- 1/3 cup cucumber
- 1 cup whole wheat noodles

Directions:

- ✓ Get a mixing bowl and put 1 cup of tomato sauce, 2/3 cup olive oil mayonnaise, 2/3 cup organic BBQ Sauce into it.
- ✓ Get a separate bowl out, then chop and dice the cucumber, tomato, red pepper, celery, kale, and spinach. Put it into a bowl.
- ✓ Take 1 cup of raw Whole Wheat Noodles and boil them on the element at medium-high. Cook for 45 minutes then turn the stove down to low for 15 minutes.

- ✓ Put the sauces into a saucepan and heat it up, then add the veggie mixture and the noodles. Once they are cooked all the way through, put then into the chilli and stir it on low heat for 10 minutes.

Snacks – Almonds, peanuts, cashews, pecans, walnuts, seeds, apple, kiwi, mango, orange.

Lunch – Chicken salad, quinoa salmon and small salad, fruit salad, grilled tofu, veggies, ham or turkey sandwich, vegetarian veggie soup.

Dinner – Veggie burger, tofu hot dog, veggie stir fry, potato salad, lean beef and whole wheat noodles.

Warning/Attention

Before you start this workout program make sure you consult with your physician. Stop exercising if you feel pain, faint, dizziness or shortness of breath.

It is always important to consult your physician before starting an exercise program. This is particularly true if any of the following apply to your current medical condition:

- Chest pain or pain in the neck and/or arm
- Shortness of breath
- A diagnosed heart condition
- Joint and/or bone problems
- Currently taking cardiac and/or blood pressure medications
- Have not previously been physically active
- Dizziness

If none of these apply to you, start gradually and sensibly.

However, if you feel any of the physical symptoms listed above when you start your exercise program, contact your physician right away.

If one or more of the statements listed above applies for you, see your physician before beginning an exercise program. An exercise – stress test may be used to help plan your exercise program.

Chapter 20 ~ Exercises

Core Stability Training:
45 seconds work/10 seconds rest

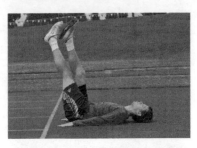

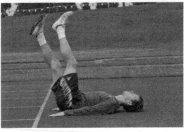

Wide Scissor

- o Lower back into the ground
- o Lift the legs up to the sky
- o Cross your leg and contract your inner thighs while using your core

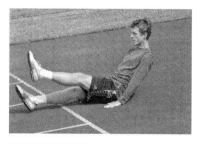

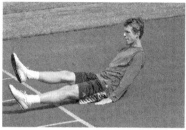

Flutter Kicks

- Hand to the side of your gluts
- Lift your legs about 6 inches off the ground
- Lean back to a 45-degree angle
- Alternate your legs, lifting up and down
- Keep your core engaged

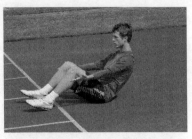

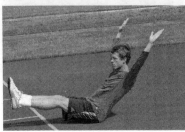

V- Hold

- First position: heels down and hands at the knees

- Lean slightly back, tuck hips under

- Second position: legs up 6 inches and arms behind your head

- Abs in tight and strong, head up and looking forward

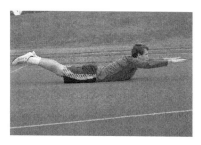

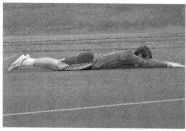

Superman

- First lay flat on your stomach
- Lift your chest up off the ground
- Make sure your head is looking forward
- Raise legs and arms
- Core engaged and in tight

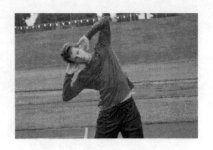

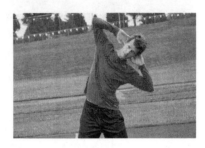

Standing Oblique Crunches

- Think about a bar going through your hips, hips stationary
- Hand slightly on your head and keep your elbows out
- Move hips laterally from side to side
- Keep abs tight

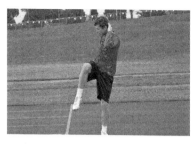
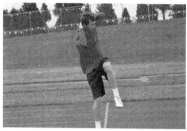

Standing Cross Abdominal Crunch

- Opposite elbow to the opposite knee
- Core engaged
- Twist your torso

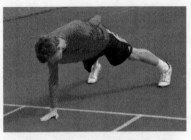

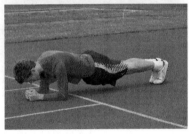

Single Arm Plank/Elbow Plank

- Legs straight and on the toes
- For elbow plank, keep your arms at a 90-degree angle
- For a Single arm plank, keep your elbow, wrist and shoulder in line with one another
- Back flat
- Core engaged
- Single arm plank: hold 30 seconds each arm

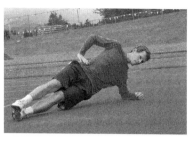

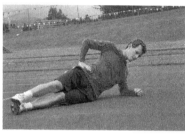

Side Plank Hip Raise

- Stack your feet on top of one another
- Elbow at a 90-degree angle, and the other hand on the hip
- Raise and lower your hips
- Core is engaged
- Push your shoulder away from your neck

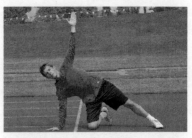
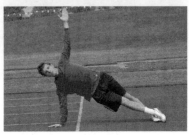

Side Plank

- Hand on the ground, wrist, elbow and shoulder inline other hand in the air
- Stack your feet on top of one another
- Raise your hips up and push your shoulder away from your neck
- Core engaged

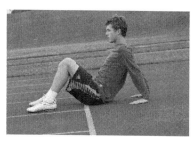

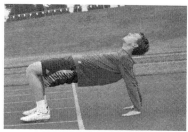

Reverse Tabletop

- Feet flat on the ground, hands facing your feet
- Raise your hips up high to the sky
- From the knees to the chest, keep flat, like a table
- Don't throw your neck back

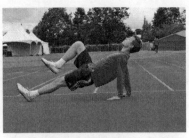

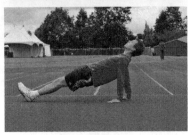

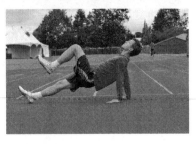

Reverse Mountain Climbers

- o   Hand faces your heels
- o   Straight line from the head to feet
- o   Raise one knee to your chest
- o   Shoulders, elbows and wrist inline
- o   Abs in tight

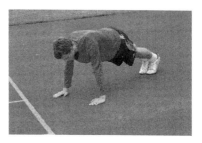

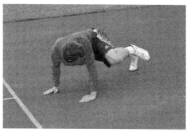

Push-Up Abs

- Back is flat
- Shoulders, elbow and wrist inline
- Head in neutral spine
- Knee to shoulder
- Slight twist in your torso, abs engaged

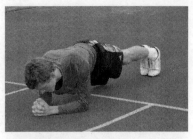

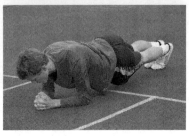

Plank Hip Twist

- Shoulders over elbows
- Arms at a 90 degree angle
- Twist your hips left to right
- Legs straight
- Head in neutral spine
- Core in tight
- Back is flat

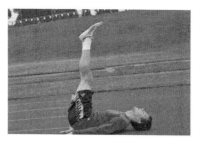
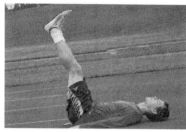

Lower Abs Leg Lift

- Lower back pressed into the ground
- Legs up to the sky
- Lift your hips up off the ground and then lower slowly
- Relax your neck and keep your core engaged
- Press your hands to the ground beside your gluts

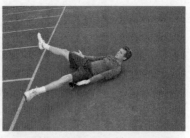

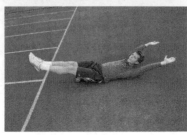

Jumping Jack Abs

- Press your lower back into the ground
- Lift your shoulder blades and chest off the ground
- Leg lifted up, arms up
- Do a jumping jack motion, hands and legs go to the side then back to center
- Core in tight and strong

Cardiovascular Interval Training

Interval: 45 seconds/15 seconds rest

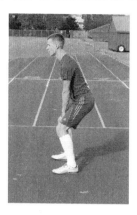 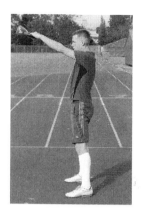

Kettle Bell Swing

- Slight bend at the knees
- Arms are loose, don't use arm strength
- Use power from the hip as you straighten your legs
- Core in tight
- Chest up, head up and look forward
- Body weight in the gluts and heels

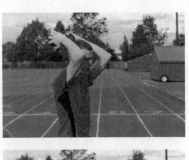

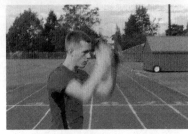

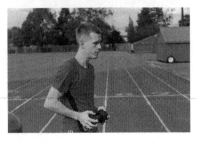

Weight Slam Down

- o   Hands on either side of the weight
- o   Pull the weight down in front of you
- o   Bottom elbows to ribs, weight to hips

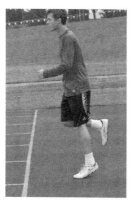

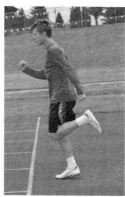

Jogging In Place

- Get your heels up to the butt
- Fast pace up and down
- Hands on hips or brush them to your ribs
- Core engaged

Strength Training

3 sets: 20 reps

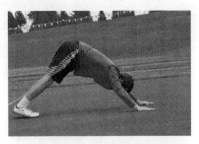

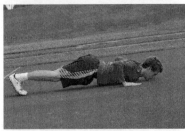

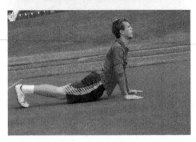

Dive Bomber

- Downward, chest to quads, heels down and hands wide
- Drive the head down and skim the chest on the ground
- On tops of the toes, chest up and pelvis to the floor
- Core engaged

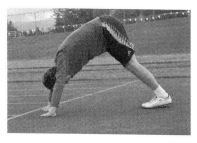

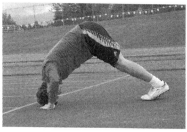

Downward Dog Shoulder Press

- Hips up to the sky
- Heels drive down
- Fingers facing each other, head down and up
- Abs in strong and tight
- Chest to the quads

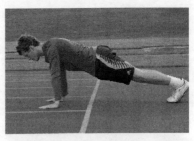

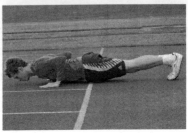

Push-Ups

- Back is flat
- Elbows beside the ribcage, and chest to the ground
- Neck in neutral spine
- Straight legs
- Core in tight and active

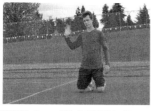 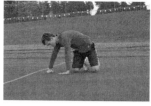
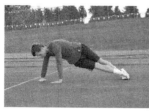 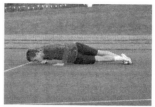

Side Push Up:

- From your knees, put your hands on the ground and make an L shape with your hands
- Feet are stacked on top of one another
- Hand closest to me elbow goes into the ribcage and the other elbow goes out
- Slight twist in the torso as you lower your oblique's to the floor and up
- Abs engaged

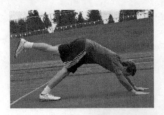
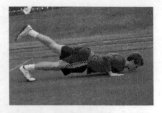
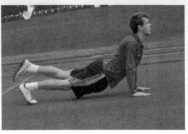

Single Leg Dive Bomber Push-Up:

- In a downward dog position, lift one leg high up to the sky
- Bend the elbows and drive the chest to the ground then come up
- Lift the leg up off the ground, pelvis to the ground and chest facing forward
- Press your shoulders away from your neck
- Core engaged

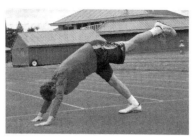

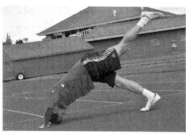

Single Leg Shoulder Press:

- Leg up to the sky
- Hips are inline
- Elbows bend to the outside and head down
- Core tight
- Keep the leg on the ground straight and the heel down

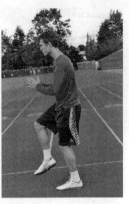

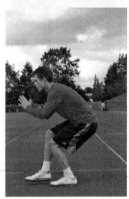

Single Leg Squat

- Keep the knee of the leg on the ground over your foot
- Gluts shoot to the back of the room
- Back is flat
- Leg off the ground
- Core in tight
- Chest up slightly

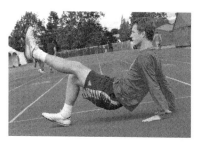

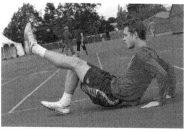

Single Leg Triceps Dip

- Knees in line with each other and lift one leg up
- Bend the elbows to the back and lower the hips to the ground
- Abs engaged
- Focus forward

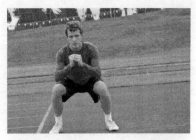

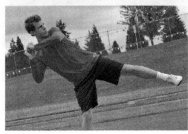

Squat with Side Kick

- o Legs at a 90-degree angle
- o Chest up, hands in front
- o Hips in line with one another
- o Bend laterally then kick to the side
- o Core in tight
- o Back is flat

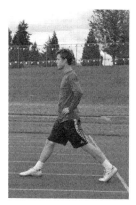

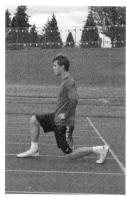

Stationary Lunge

- Toes pointed forward
- Front leg knee over ankle
- Back leg hip over knee
- Chest up
- Back is flat
- Core engaged

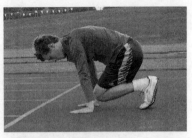
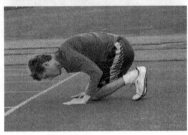

Triceps Ball

- Shoulders over your wrist
- On the top your toes, knees an inch away from the ground
- Elbows to the ribcage and, pointed back
- Core engaged

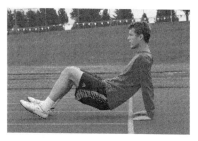
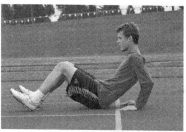

Triceps Dips

- Heels down on the ground
- Lift the hips off the ground
- Bend the elbows to the back
- Core engaged

Stretches and Yoga Poses:

Hold Stretch: 1 minute each side

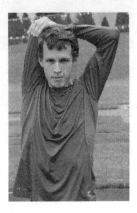

Triceps Stretch

- o Elbow to the side of the head
- o Slightly pull the elbow back to feel the stretch

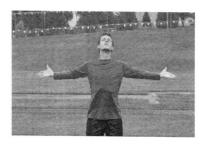

Chest Stretch

- Head slightly tilted up to the sky
- Slight arch in the back
- Chest up to the sky and arms out, thumbs point to the back

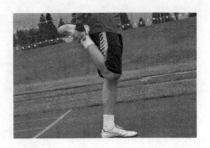

Quadriceps Stretch

- o   Hand grabs the ankle and keep your knees inline
- o   Push the hip out
- o   Chest up and centre
- o   Keep the whole foot flat on the ground

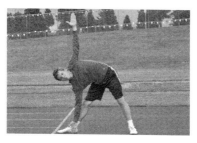

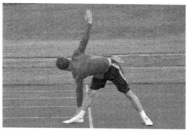

Triangle/Twisting Triangle

- One leg point forward the other leg pointed to the side
- Hand on the ground, shin, or knee, and the other hand to the sky
- Hips in line with one another
- Look forward or up to the top hand

Twisting Triangle

- Opposite hand to the leg and twist the spine
- Reach the opposite hand up to the sky

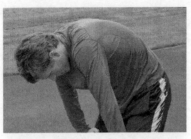

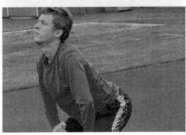

Cat/Cow Pose

- Slight bend in the knee
- Hands on your quadriceps
- Round the back and put the chin to the chest
- Arch the back and look up

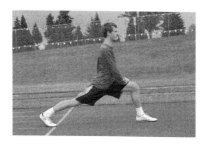

Hip Flexor Stretch

- Back leg straight on top of the toes
- Front leg at a 90-degree angle
- Hand on the front quad
- Chest up
- Drive the hips down towards the front heel

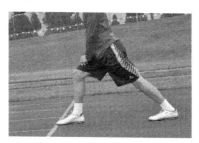

Calf Stretch

- Front leg bent slightly
- Hands on the front quad
- Back leg straight and heel down on the ground

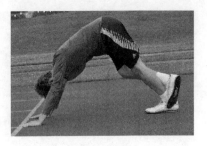

Downward Dog Calf Stretch

- Hip high to the sky
- Drive your chest to the quads
- Straight arms, press shoulders away from the ears
- Cross one leg over the other while the other heel is on the ground

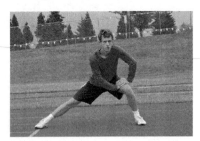

Side Lunge Stretch

- Keep one leg over the foot
- Other leg is straight and feel the stretch in the inner thigh
- Hand on your quad to support your lower back
- Chest up and back in neutral spine

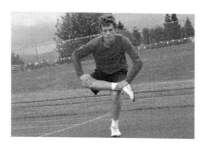

Gluteus Maximus Stretch

- Cross your ankle over the opposite knee
- The knee of the foot that is on the ground is over your foot
- Lower the hips and sit into the squat
- Chest up and back flat
- Core engaged

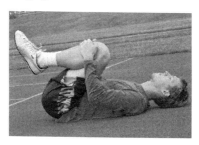

Knee Hug

- Press your lower back into the ground
- Head on the floor
- Grab your knees and pull them into your chest
- Core engaged

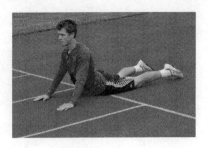

Cobra

- Pelvis on the floor
- Top of the feet on the floor
- Straight arms and chest up
- Look forward

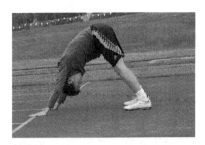

Downward Dog

- Hands are wide and pressing away from the head
- Chest driving toward the quads
- Press the heels down toward the floor
- Hips are high to the sky
- Head in-between your arms

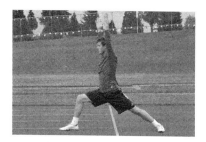

Warrior 1

- Front leg 90 degree angle
- Back leg straight outside of the foot pressing into the floor
- Hip forward
- Arm straight & shoulders away from your ears
- Palms facing each other

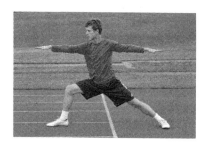

Warrior 2

- Hips in line with one another
- Front foot pressed into the ground
- Front leg at a 90 degree angle
- Chest up
- Arms lengthened out and focus forward

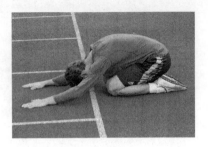

Child's Pose

- o Butt to your heel
- o Chest to quads
- o Arm straight over head

Workout Plan:

Monday: 25 minute power walk, strength

Tuesday: Yoga/ stretch +3, 10 min slow walk

Wednesday: Cardio*2, strength, core stability

Thursday: Power Walk 25 min, core stability

Friday: Rest

Saturday: Core stability, yoga

Sunday: Rest/ or stretch

Chapter 21 ~ Myths of Fitness

I want to explain there are millions of diet and fitness gimmicks out there that want to steal your money and you need to know what's real and what's fake in the fitness industry.

I have a heart for people and want to get you what you deserve. You deserve to hear the truth that people will make up something on the spot and make it look really professional to get your money and not achieve the results, (for example: a celebrity magic weight loss pill).

You may get mad and frustrated with your body and the products because you may not know what's right or wrong.

First, I want to say if you hear any diet/nutrition book that says you need to go on a diet or take out an important food group like fats, protein or carbs ignore everything they tell you.

Diets don't work, nutrition is a lifestyle. That's why I don't like to use the word diet. Don't go on a carb diet or just eat carbs and protein because this is not healthy.

We need healthy fats, proteins and carbs as all of these have benefits to a healthy life and these all give nourishment to your muscles and bones.

If you start a diet that neglects important food groups you will start to feel sluggish, sleepy, low on energy, and fatigued. It can mess up your whole daily balance.

I want to help guide you away from all the myths out there. Okay, women this one is for you, the myth is: if women lift weights, they will get bulky/husky? That answer is no.

If you use 5lbs or 10lbs you won't build bulky muscle. It's not realistic to get big on 5 or 10lbs. You need to lift heavy weight and drink protein powder/protein foods to gain muscle weight.

Lifting light weights will improve your overall bodily strength and conditioning. It is possible to increase strength without gaining mass.

By lifting light weights, you are improving you own body weight strength. So ladies, you won't get big if you use low weights like 5-10lbs.

Myth: If you don't have time or don't put enough effort into working out it's not worth it? My answer would be that this is an excuse to skip physical activity.

We have time and we can do something active during the day. Go for a walk, run, play on the playground with your kids, play sports.

It's a lifestyle not a finish line. Let me ask you, is your health worth it means you get to see your kids grow up?

Is it worth it if it results in living a long healthy life and growing old with your spouse? Is it worth it to have more time with your friends?

If you think it's not worth it, then you will miss out on what the future has in store for you. New friends, adventures and journeys.

My opinion is that it is worth it to spend the time and effort to make sure I have good health and have a fun life. Yes, it's totally worth every single penny and minute in the gym.

Myth: I can get a six pack by doing just abs crunches. This is a big topic that lots of people ask about. People always ask me about how they can get a six pack or flat stomach.

The short answer is that you need to burn that fat off your stomach before you can start showing your abs. This means that you need to do cardiovascular training along with core interval training.

You have to do both at the same time. Do cardio and abs to work multiple muscles and burn fat and build abdominal strength. Get that down pat and get your abs ready for the beach.

Truth: Can fitness reduce the chance of getting sick? Yes it can, I'll explain. The average adult who is healthy should only get sick 1-4 times a year. There are ways to reduce sickness in your body.

Step 1: Clean up and wash your hands and body daily.

Step 2: Boost your immune system through exercise, minerals and vitamins.

Step 3: Meditate and relax 5-10 minutes a day to clear your stress and mind and calm yourself down to get back to your normal state.

Step 4: Sleep well and avoid fast food and junk food.

All of these things can improve your overall health and reduce sickness. Yes, health and wellness can reduce sickness.

Myth: Pregnant women can't do abs crunches. My first advice is to get clearance from your doctor before starting any fitness program.

From my own perspective, it is beneficial for the mom and the baby to strengthen her core during pregnancy. It will help during the pregnancy and labour process of the birth.

Core stability and strength is good. It's okay to do crunches, but not a lot, try to stick with standing abdominal work. Avoid lying on your back to avoid any oxygen problems for the baby or raising the mom's blood pressure during her last trimester.

In the last trimester, don't do crunches, but until then it is okay. Pregnant women need to stay active during pregnancy.

Watch your nutrition during the months of pregnancy so you don't fill your baby up with anything that can damage its lungs, organs, heart or kidneys.

Your personal trainer should guide you and monitor you. Go at your own pace and don't push yourself to any limits.

Myth: You can't work out when you are old and stiff. In the end, age doesn't define if you can work out, your flexibility does.

Flexibility determines how old you are. If your spine is flexible you are young and if it's stiff and inflexible you are old.

For those who are stiff, I would say their options are to get an effective workout. Aqua fit classes take the pain off your joints and help you get a good workout in the water without feeling any pain.

So, no, age doesn't matter because you can still do yoga and aqua fit to get stronger and more mobile.

We may use our age as excuses for not working out. That's ridiculous. What if you're young and have a bad back? You can still work out, even if it is just chair aerobics.

Myth: If you're not sweating you're not achieving results. If you are moving more today than yesterday, you are one step closer to your goal then before.

Sweat is important to open up your pores and get unwanted fat and salts out of your body. If you walked more today than yesterday that's all that matters.

You will achieve your results in time. The answer is you don't have to sweat all the time to lose weight, lose inches or achieve results.

Myth: You should wait to eat until you're hungry. If we all did that we would just overdo it and fill our stomach with unhealthy things.

Sometimes we think we are hungry, but we are just dehydrated. You need to eat a healthy breakfast in the morning even if you are not hungry.

Drink a small smoothie to get some nutrient-dense foods into your body for fuel and energy. Our culture doesn't always know what hungry is because we have all the food we need.

We need to fill up on healthy foods so we won't feel disgusted about unhealthy choices that will put our systems in a stage of denial because of what we consumed. Eat five small meals or three medium meals a day.

Myth: You don't need to count calories to lose weight. The truth is you need to know what you are consuming so you can count how many calories you are going to need to burn to lose weight.

If you eat more than you burn, you will not lose weight. People think that they don't need to have a food journal or count calories, but the truth is that you need to train your eye to know what a serving size looks like and how many calories are in a portion for one person.

The answer is that you need to know your calorie intake and outtake for workout and nutrition purposes to achieve weight loss goals.

Chapter 22 ~ Benefits/Tips on Fitness

I am going to tell you a lot of benefits that come with fitness. It isn't all about big biceps or six-pack abs. There is so much more than just that. You're thinking, why would he say that?

Because fitness deals with more than just the physical, it involves the emotional, mental and spiritual barriers in your life. Okay, so let me start with some of the small facts about fitness, and then work my way up to the more complex and mind-blowing ones.

First, exercise helps with your physical goals like weight loss, muscular hypertrophy and muscular endurance.

Cardiovascular fitness can help reduce the amount of fat that is on your body. Fitness in general speeds up your metabolism so that you can burn calories faster. Your metabolism will be even faster if you drink a nice big glass of water in the morning.

Strength training is beneficial to sculpt muscles and get them showing after you burn that fat off during the cardio session.

Fitness can help regulate your blood pressure.

Drinking 8-12 medium size glasses a day can help with your skin, metabolism.

Getting a six-pack doesn't come from doing crunches, it comes when you burn that fat off your body through fast body movement. Six-packs are made in the kitchen not gym.

When you move your upper body and lower body you burn more calories than from just isolating one muscle.

Did you know that your legs muscles (Gluteus, Hamstrings, Quadriceps, adductors, and abductors) are the largest muscles in your body? When you start moving your largest muscle group you go into a fat burning zone.

Fitness can be used to help break through emotional barrier. When your trainer says that you should leave all your emotions, anger, frustrations and sadness in the gym, you will leave changed.

By using a physical obstacle, it can challenge you to deal with your emotions in a healthy way by talking and shouting, screaming, etc. Let all that pain go and smash through that wall.

The benefits of mental strength are more important than you think. For example, if I tell you to do a lunge with a bicep curl, you need to focus on the moment and not think about the person beside you.

I guarantee you will hurt yourself eventually if you lose focus. Once you lose your focus on what you are doing, you might move in a direction you didn't want to go in the first place.

When you work out, think about the muscle you are working on and control it. Think about the form, safety, and technique.

Fitness is 80% mental and 20% physical. The reason is that when you get sore or tired during that workout you need to dig deep inside your head and push through that burn, and once you keep going and don't stop, that's when the change will happen.

When you are sore it's a sign that you pushed yourself to the limits and are getting stronger. Don't think that just because you aren't sore you didn't get a great workout.

It's like when people feel that fiery burn in their legs or arms they stop. That burn in your muscles is burning up the fat and calories you ate before you worked out. That burn is key to losing weight or burning fat or calories.

Fitness helps deal with bad habits like stress eating or other personal problems. You need to understand that when you see yourself grabbing for food every few minutes you need to catch yourself and acknowledge your behavior and snap it in the butt.

A fitness trainer can help you use fitness as a counsellor and overcome obstacles in your personal life and become a new person after you deal with it face to face.

The benefit of group fitness is that if you are struggling the entire team can help you through it and motivate you to do better. It's all about supporting one another and loving one another.

Aquatic fitness helps you to get an effective workout without the stress or pressure on your knees, ankles, hips or shoulders. There is no excuse not to workout. Aquatic fitness helps strengthen your muscles. It's great for athletes who have pain in their body. When you're in the water you don't feel the pain.

Fitness can help reduce your cholesterol level.

The benefit of fitness is that there is a hormone in your body that gets released when you work out that makes you feel happy and joyful. It helps you think encouraging and positive thoughts.

Cardio exercise like running, walking, jogging or doing a cardio class can help with depression.

Regular physical activity can reduce stress, improve mental power and improve your energy level.

There is 24 hours in a day which you spend about 8 hours at work and about 8 hours sleeping. North Americans spend about 5-10 hours in front of a screen. You have the power to work out or be active. Don't tell me that you don't have time when you watch three hours of TV in the evening. You can do 15-30 minutes of exercise in your home. Get a support system to keep you on track.

Fitness can build new relationships.

Exercise can help with diseases like type 2 diabetes. Nutrition and exercise can reverse it. It can even help you to get off fibre pills, which you may not need when you work out. It puts more money in your pocket instead of the pharmacy.

Exercise helps with your sports performance and attaining your goals.

Exercise can help with your sleeping pattern. When you exercise, it can help you fall asleep faster and deeper. Regular physical activity will help you sleep better.

5 Main Benefits of Healthy Nutrition

Heart Health

Lower your cholesterol by eating less consumption of saturated fats and trans-fat foods like fried food, fatty oils, margarine, and red meat.

These can increase your cholesterol level. We need to avoid these in our daily nutrition. Instead, eat 2-3 servings of fresh veggies, fruits and whole grains.

Bone and Strength

Getting calcium and dairy products into your system can help you get strong bones and healthy teeth. Many people can get osteoporosis from a lack of calcium in the first 30 years of growing up.

There are ways to prevent osteoporosis, such as regular physical activity, taking supplements and eating dairy products throughout the day.

Getting more Vitamin A, D, and K into your diet is very important. 90 percent of calcium is found in your teeth and bones and 10 percent is found in your blood stream.

We need to be cautious and aware of our intake and outtake of these supplements. To take care of your body, you need to make sure your teeth and bones are healthy and strong throughout your life.

Energy

It was found that people who feel sluggish and tired all the time are not getting enough energy to last them through the whole day.

The good news is that there are several ways to increase the amount of energy you have every day. Regular exercise can increase the endorphin hormone levels in your body.

Better heart health can help boost endurance throughout your day. Improve your sleeping pattern and choose to exercise to increase the endorphins that strengthen your heart and improve stamina during your workout.

Brain Health

Here are a few foods that will help with brain function and stability at any age. Brain health improving foods are blueberries, wild salmon, nuts, seeds, avocado and whole grains.

So as you age keep these foods in your nutrition plan that will help you function and to think better. It will help with memory and slow down the memory loss process and help you to think just as fast as you did when you were younger.

Weight Control

The first step to success is having the mindset of treating yourself with care and love. After that you need to focus on good healthy meals and looking at the recipe plan I have provided, or another recipe plan if you prefer.

The second step is to have a good heart pumping workout, especially focusing on toning exercises like bodily resistance.

Closing ~ Lifesaver

All these segments have been a time to reflect on the direction of success. I will help you as your personal trainer, being a light in this messed up world.

I pray and hope that all these tips and advice will help you now and in the future. Share my encouragement with your family and friends.

Let them know that we are all in this together and no one is left behind on this journey. We all know people who could use that extra boost of encouragement and use that to motivate them to get up and get going.

This is not just a onetime deal, if you finish this program or fitness counselling session, always come back for more if you need that extra help when all seems hopeless.

I want to be that trainer who is going to do whatever it takes to challenge you and help you with your feelings and emotions and change your life. I want to be your mentor and counsellor.

I love you guys and care for your safety and health. If you want to follow me on social media, my username is "Braydon's Fitness" on Facebook, Twitter, YouTube, Tumblr, Instagram and Pinterest.

I would love to help keep you on track and do what I can to encourage you and keep you going.

Made in the USA
Charleston, SC
12 August 2016